Hand Book of
MEAT SCIENCE

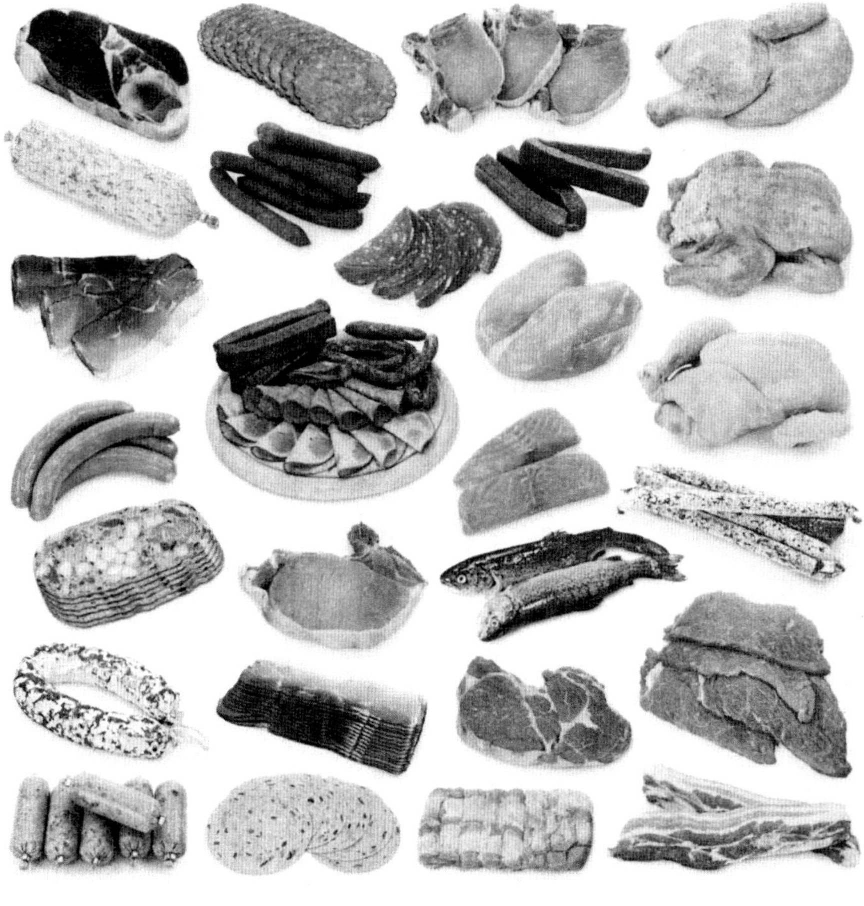

Hand Book of
MEAT SCIENCE

Authors

Prabhat Kumar Mandal
Associate Professor
Department of Livestock Products Technology
Rajiv Gandhi Institute of Veterinary
Education and Research, Kurumbapet
Puducherry-605009
e-mail : mandalpkm@gmail.com

Ashim Kumar Biswas
Senior Scientist (LPT)
Division of Post-Harvest Technology, ICAR-CARI,
Izatnagar, Bareilly-243122 (U.P.)
e-mail: biswaslpt@gmail.com

SSPH

SATISH SERIAL PUBLISHING HOUSE
403, Express Tower, Commercial Complex
Azadpur, Delhi-110033 (India)
Phone : 011-27672852, Fax : 91-11-27672046
e-mail : info@satishserial.com, hkjain1975@yahoo.com
Website : www.satishserial.com

Published by :

SATISH SERIAL PUBLISHING HOUSE
403, Express Tower, Commercial Complex, Azadpur, Delhi-110033 (INDIA)
Phone : 011-27672852 Fax : 91-11-27672046
E-mail : info@satishserial.com, hkjain1975@yahoo.com

ISBN 978-93-86200-41-9 (HB)

Composed, Designed & Printed in India

About the Authors

Dr. Prabhat Kumar Mandal was born in 1967 in West Bengal, got BVSc. & A.H. from Bidhan Chandra Krishi Viswavidyalaya, Kolkata, in 1991 and did his MVSc & Ph.D majoring in Livestock Products Technology from Indian Veterinary Research Institute, Izatnagar in the year 1993 and 1996, respectively. He is a recipient of National Scholarship from GOI (1984-1991), JRF (1991–1993) and SRF (1993–1996) from IVRI. He worked for a short period (1996) as Scientist (ARS) in ICAR and then joined as Assistant Professor in Dept of LPT in September 1996, in Rajiv Gandhi College of Veterinary and Animal Sciences, Pondicherry. He was promoted as Associate Professor in March, 2005 and Associate Professor, Senior Grade from March, 2008.

Dr. Mandal is teaching several UG and PG courses related to Livestock Products Technology and engaged in research on Meat Science and Technology more than 20 years. His research achievements include development of chicken meat balls from spent hen meat, utilization of blood protein isolates in sausages and cakes, development of poultry products utilizing edible byproducts, low fat restructured chicken block using gizzard and natural preservatives. Presently he is working on development of functional meat foods with natural preservatives. Dr. Mandal has more than 150 publications to his credit.

He worked as Visiting Professor in Hankyong National Univrsity, South Korea and Konkuk University, Seoul from March, 2008 to February, 2010. He was Associate Editor/Editor, Journal of Meat Science published by IMSA since 2003 -13. Presently Dr. Mandal is Chief Editor of International Journal of Meat Science, Journal of Meat Science and Journal of Food & Nutrition Research. He has edited an advance reference book "Animal Products Technology" and Co-author of books "Poultry, Egg and Fish Processing Technology" for PG level and "Abattoir, Byproducts and Wool" for U. G. Veterinary students and "Practical Meat Science". Dr. Mandal is a Fellow of Indian Poultry Science Association and Indian Meat Science Association.

Dr. Ashim Kumar Biswas Born on 05th March 1978 in West Bengal, got BVSc. & A.H. from WBUA& FSc, Kolkata in 2000, MVSc. (in 2002) and Ph.D (in 2005) in Livestock Products Technology from, Indian Veterinary Research Institute, Izatnagar. In 2005, he joined as Assistant Professor in the Department of LPT, SKUAST-Jammu. On Feb 2007, he joined as Assistant Professor in the Department of LPT, GADVASU, Ludhiana. Presently he is serving as Senior Scientist in Division of Post-Harvest

Technology at Central Avian Research Institute (ICAR), Izatnagar. He has more than 150 publications to his credit.

His main achievements in research is relating to evaluation of export buffalo meat for quality, development of enrobed meat products, restructured buffalo meat blocks, functional based & shelf stable value added meat products. His research also focused on development and validation of HPLC methodologies for detection of pesticide and veterinary drug residues in meat and meat products. He also standardized molecular techniques (PCR) for the detection of bacterial pathogens in livestock products. He teaches several LPT courses at the University and guides many undergraduate and postgraduate students since 2006. He handled or currently handling several research projects and grants funded by MFPI, DST, RKVY (Govt. of India), ICAR, etc. in the capacity of PI and Co-PI.

He has Co-edited an advance reference book "Animal Products Technology" and author of a text book "Poultry, Egg and Fish Processing Technology" for PG level and another text book "Abattoir, Byproducts and Wool" for U. G Veterinary students and "Practical Meat Science". Dr. Biswas is a fellow of Indian Poultry Science Association, NAAS Associate, Associate Editor, Journal of Meat Science and Indian Journal of Poultry Science.

Preface

Foods of animal origin with high biological value are very important source of animal proteins and other important nutrients for life sustenance of human being. There is heavy demand for the muscle foods and the consumers are very much aware about the health benefits of muscle foods. Accordingly lots of research and developments are going on in this area to provide quality meat and meat products. India, is experiencing rapid growth in animal and poultry industry especially in meat industry. Presently, India ranks 5th in meat and poultry production in the world.

Recently, the Veterinary Council of Indian has revised the curriculum for undergraduate (BVSc&AH) study and the course contents are thoroughly revised under "Minimum Standard of Veterinary Educations" (MSVE) Regulations, 2016. Under the department of Livestock Products Technology one of the important portions in the syllabus is Meat Science (Unit-4). However, at present no proper text book is available covering this course for the ready reference of the students. We both have been teaching the earlier course from the beginning of the VCI syllabus, hence, we felt a book covering the new syllabus with a easy reading is very much necessary for the students. A hand book is one which deals with the basic information about a subject. This book is designed for easy understanding of the subject with precise points, especially for the students. The syllabus on Meat Science is covered under 17 topics, each to be covered in one lecture. The topics are presented in a very easy language with précised points, figures, tables and charts. We hope this Handbook will be very much useful to the under graduate students of veterinary and animal sciences, and teachers who are engaged in teaching students.

Prabhat Kumar Mandal
Ashim Kumar Biswas

Contents

1

Prospect of Meat Industry in India

India is having largest livestock resources in the world. Presently, India produces about 6.6 million MT of meat, ranking fifth in the world. The low meat production is due to lower productivity coupled with low slaughter rate.

Table 1. Livestock population and meat production in India

Species	Population (Million)	Percentage (To world)	Qty of meat (000 MT)	Rank
Cattle	175	12.7	0.88	Second
Buffalo	105	56.7	1.43	First
Sheep	65	6.0	0.24	Third
Goat	126	14.5	0.48	Second
Pigs	13.84	1.47	0.48	-
Chicken	1814	3.2	2.02	Fifth
Duck	35	3.0	-	Fifth

FAO, 2009

Livestock Economy

- Livestock farming in India has a pivotal role in rural economy, employment and foreign exchange earnings.
- The contribution of livestock sector to the total GDP has remained steady in the past few years.
- The value of output from livestock sector is 1, 64, 509 crores, which is 29.95% of agricultural GDP and 4.3% of national GDP.
- The value output of meat group is 24,876 crores, milk group 1,07,544 crores, egg group 5, 238 crores and poultry group 10, 627 crores.

Table 2. Meat production in India (,000 tonnes)

Species	1975	1985	1995	2005	2010
Beef & veal	71	89	1,292	924	880
Buffalo meat	117	135	1,204	1348	1430
Mutton	117	135	179	230	239
Goat meat	-	417	474	475	531
Pork	269	315	420	472	480
Poultry meat	156	85	578	549	2026
Total*	**821**	**1236**	**4,272**	**4312**	**6316**

* including meat from other species

Slaughterhouses/Meat Plants

- Majority of the slaughterhouses are traditional type lacking adequate facilities
- Animals are slaughtered and dressed on open ground without any care of clean meat production.
- Carcasses are exposed to heavy contamination from dung and soil.
- No ante mortem and post mortem inspection and clandestine slaughter practices.
- There are about 3,600 recognized slaughterhouses, 10 modern abattoirs, 6 bacon factories and 170 small meat processing units under MFPO license.
- In the fourth five year plan (1966-72) eight modern bacon factories for pork processing were established.
- These bacon factories are situated in Haringhata (West Bengal), Ranchi (Jharkhand), Alwar (Rajasthan), Gannavaram (Andhra Pradesh), Ernakulum (Kerala) and Mumbai (Maharashtra).
- First modern slaughterhouse established at Deonar (near Mumbai) in 1971 slaughtering nearly 500 large animals and 7-10 thousands sheep and goat per day.
- In 1978-79, 1982 and 1984 three other slaughterhouses has been set up by the Ministry of Agriculture at Aurangabad (Maharashtra), Usagaon (Goa) and Durgapur (West Bengal).

- A modern abattoir at CFTRI is involved in training butchers, veterinarians and meat technologists.
- Presently India has more than twenty modern meat plants for export.

Meat Export

- Export is mainly as live animals (17%), meat (82%), dairy products and eggs (1%).
- At global level India's export and import accounts for only 0.17 per cent of each.
- The meat for export has to pass through stringent inspection of A.M./P.M. examination.
- Dressed carcasses are chilled, deboned and packed into different cuts and frozen (-40 °C) for export.
- Indian meat (buffalo) exports started with 2000 tonnes in the year 1973-74 and increased to about 60,000 MT in 1987-88 and 173000 MT in 1995-96.
- The Middle East countries showed rapid growth and export reached 54,582 tonnes in 1981 - 82.
- The major importing countries were UAE, Kuwait, Saudi Arabia, Oman, Bahrain, Qatar, Yemen, Malaysia, Thailand and Maldives.
- Presently major export is buffalo meat accounting 98% of total meat exports.
- India also exports processed meat to Jordan, Russia, Oman and Bahrain.
- Meat export is mostly through private modern abattoirs with Sanitary and Phyto-sanitary (SPS) measures as per OIE/WTO with HACCP, ISO-9001 certificates.

Table 3. Export of meat and meat products (Qty.: in thousand MT; Value: million)

	2008-09		2009-10		2010-11	
Product	Quantity	Value	Quantity	Value	Quantity	Value
Buffalo meat	462.7	48397.1	495.01	54806	709.4	84127
Sheep/goat meat	37.79	4933.7	52.8	7472	11.91	2531.8
Pig meat	1.118	21.7	-	-	-	105.1
Poultry products	1057.02	91.76	1016.7	3721	619.2	3013.2
Processed meat	0.86	21.05	1.24	31.9	-	210.5

Source: DGCIS Annual Export

Table 4. Value of export of meat and meat products

Year	₹ (Million)
1971-72	20.0
1981-82	800.0
1991-92	1000
2001-02	13185
2010-11	90339.1

Processed Meat

- Only 3% is of meat produced is marketed in processed form.
- India started meat processing with 220 small units, and 8 bacon factories under MFPO license in 1966-1972.
- Majority of the products marketed as cured products (50%), sausages (20%) and canned meat (20%).
- Traditional meat products including kebabs, tandoori chicken, meat curry, meat samosa, meatball (kofta), meat pickle etc.
- Regional meat products are Delhi- Nihari; Goa- Goa sausage; Himachal Pradesh-Pork pickle; Jammu & Kashmir- Nate Yakini, Gostaba, Rista; and Arunachal Pradesh-Rapka.

World Meat Scenario

- Presently Codex has 169 member countries and each country having different ethnicity and food habits.
- Per capita beef consumption is highest in Argentina followed by Uruguay.

- China, Hungary, Denmark, Austria, Germany, and Spain are leading producer of pork meat.
- Mutton, lamb and goat meat is most popular in New Zealand, Uruguay, Australia, and Greece.
- Broiler consumption is highest in USA, Hong Kong, Saudi Arabia, Israel and Canada.
- Turkey meat is most liked in Israel, France, Canada and Italy.
- Europe ranks first in world meat production and Asia the second.
- North America, Europe and Oceania contribute 60% of total meat production and 85% of total meat export.
- Europe shared 55% of meat export.
- Asia contributes only 6.5%, India's share less than 1%.

Prospects of Indian Meat Industry

- Large resources of livestock, ranking- 1st in cattle & buffalo, 3rd and 5th rank in goat and poultry production.
- Animals are generally raised in nearly organic farming systems on green fodder.
- In fact, meat from these animals is almost lean contains low fat.
- The price structure is favorable to Indian meat in international markets.
- No use of chemical pesticides, veterinary drugs, hormonal compounds etc.
- A great potential exist for exporting buffalo and chicken meat in Middle-East and South-East Asian countries.
- India has advantages exporting to these countries due to less transport cost and growing demand of lean meat.
- Buffalo meat has wide demand in world market due to lean meat and animals are raised nearly organic by grass feeding.

Major Constraints of Indian Meat Industry

1. Inadequate feeds, fodder, cereal straw etc to meet livestock's needs.

2. Early mortality, ineffective culling, selling at early age due to economic constraint.
3. Improper livestock marketing system, involvement of middle man.
4. Lack of knowledge of clean meat production, grading system in meat trade and lack of pragmatic slaughter policy.
5. Inadequate infrastructure facilities for slaughtering of animals.
6. Unregistered slaughterhouses and selling fresh meat on the same day.
7. Difficulty in getting licenses/permits to set up slaughterhouses/ meat plants.
8. Selling of meat in the domestic market without proper inspection by veterinarians.
9. Lack of awareness of value addition of meat and animal byproducts.
10. Negative attitude of public towards meat on account of socio-political reason.

Important Suggestions to Improve

1. Genetic improvement through selection, cross breeding/ETT for meat.
2. Improve supply of feed, cereal straws, agro-byproducts and fodder.
3. Increasing productivity as well as quality of meat through cost effective farming.
4. Establish rural meat processing plants in dense animal tracts.
5. Establishment of at least one carcass utilization plant in each district
6. Salvaging of male buffalo calf could increase meat production.
7. Establishment of cold chain and modern storage facilities.
8. Training and education of inspector/personels.
9. Establish national directorate on meat to promote meat industry.
10. Strengthening quality monitoring with internationally approved laboratories.

□□□

2

Structure and Organisation of Muscle

The muscle tissue is mainly consists of 300 skeletal muscle, smooth muscle associated with the intestines, blood vessels and cardiac muscle. The weight of the muscular tissue is 35 to 60 per cent of the carcass weight in sheep, cattle and pigs. Generally this proportion varies inversely with that of fatty tissue, age and plane of nutrition.

Muscle Anatomy and Morphology

- A continuum of connective tissue mainly consisting of collagen encompass the muscle and its components.
- Entire muscle is surrounded by a heavy sheath of connective tissue called **epimysium**
- From epimysium, a septa of connective tissue penetrate into the muscle, separating bundle of muscle fibre known as **perimysium,**
- A fine connective tissue framework passes further inwards to surround each muscle fibre called the **endomysium**.
- The muscle cells are long, multinucleated, called muscle fibres.
- The fibres are highly specialized structural unit of muscle, comprising 75-92% of muscle volume.
- The size of the muscle fibre bundles determines the texture of the meat.

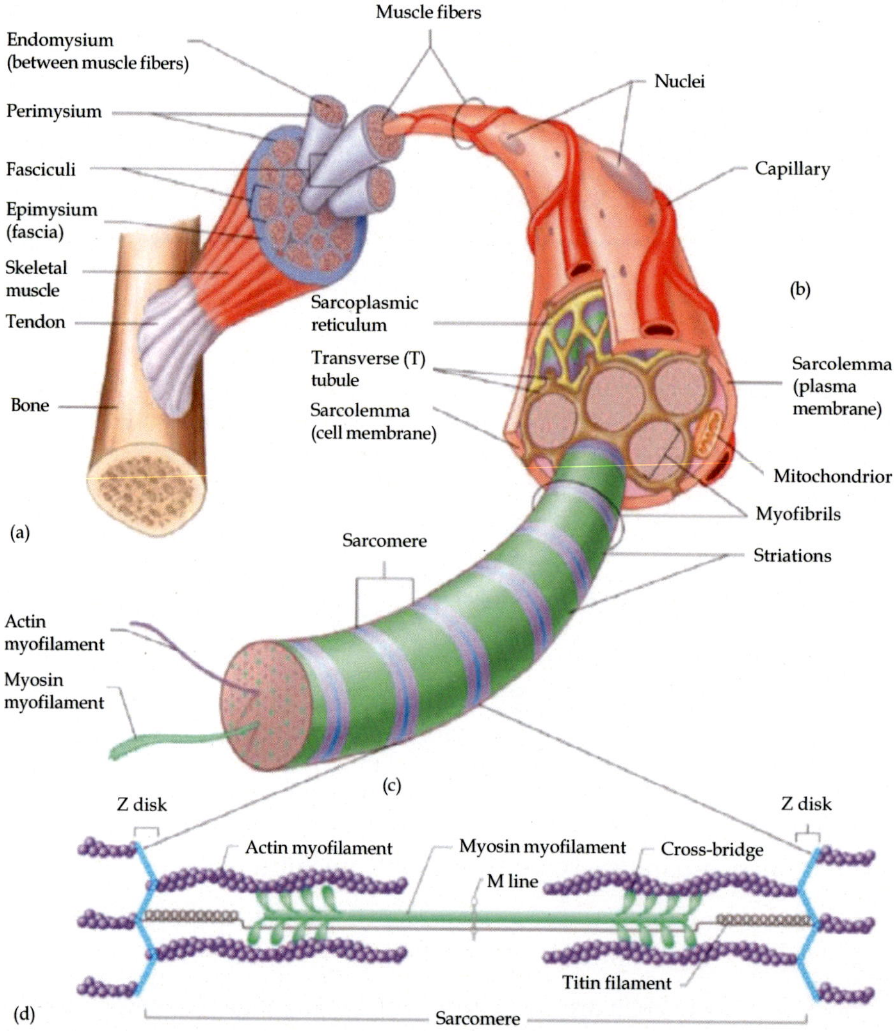

Muscle to Myofilament

Organization of Muscle Fibre

- Fibres are long, narrow, multinucleated cells extending to entire length of the muscle, with diameter of 10-100 μm.
- Each fibre underneath the endomysium, is surrounded by a membrane, known as **sarcolemma**.
- Along the length and breadth of the fibre, invaginations of the sarcolemma form a network of tubules referred to as **T system or T tubules**.

- Muscle fibre may have several hundred of nuclei located peripherally below the sarcolemma.
- Nearly 75-80 per cent of muscle fibre is organelles called **myofibrils** dipped in protoplasm like fluid known as **sarcoplasm**.
- Myofibrils are long, cylindrical tube like filaments usually 1-2 μm in diameter.
- **Myofilaments** are composed of thick and thin filaments of the myofibril.
- Thick and thin filaments are aligned parallel to each other across the entire myofibril.
- Thick and thin filaments overlap in certain portions, leading to characteristic banding or striated appearance.
- Myofibrils consisting of repeating units joined in series called **sarcomeres.**

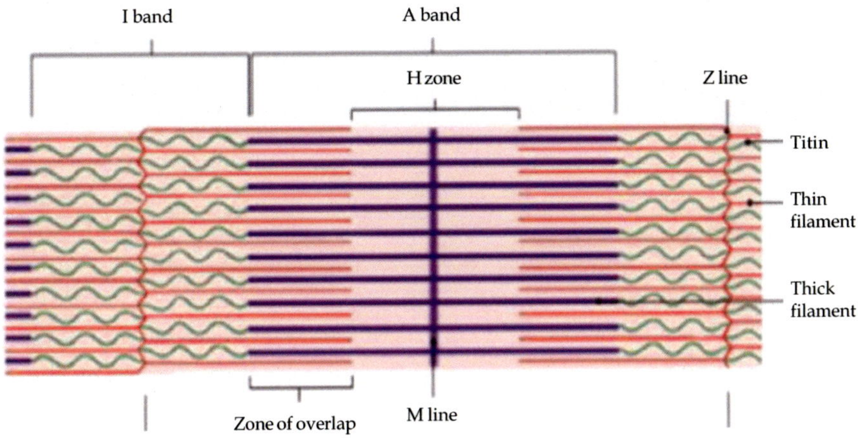

Sarcomere

Sarcomere Organization

- The repeating contractile unit of the myofibril is the sarcomere.
- It comprised of two halves of thin filaments on either side of thick filaments.
- This is the portion of the myofibril between two adjacent Z disc.

- The Z disc oriented perpendicular to the thin filaments and the long axis of the myofibril.
- The thin filaments are isotropic called I band, thick filaments are anisotropic called 'A' bands.
- In the centre of the A band, a bare zone free of these projection exists.
- The bare zone is bisected by the 'M' line, bare region is referred as 'H' zone.

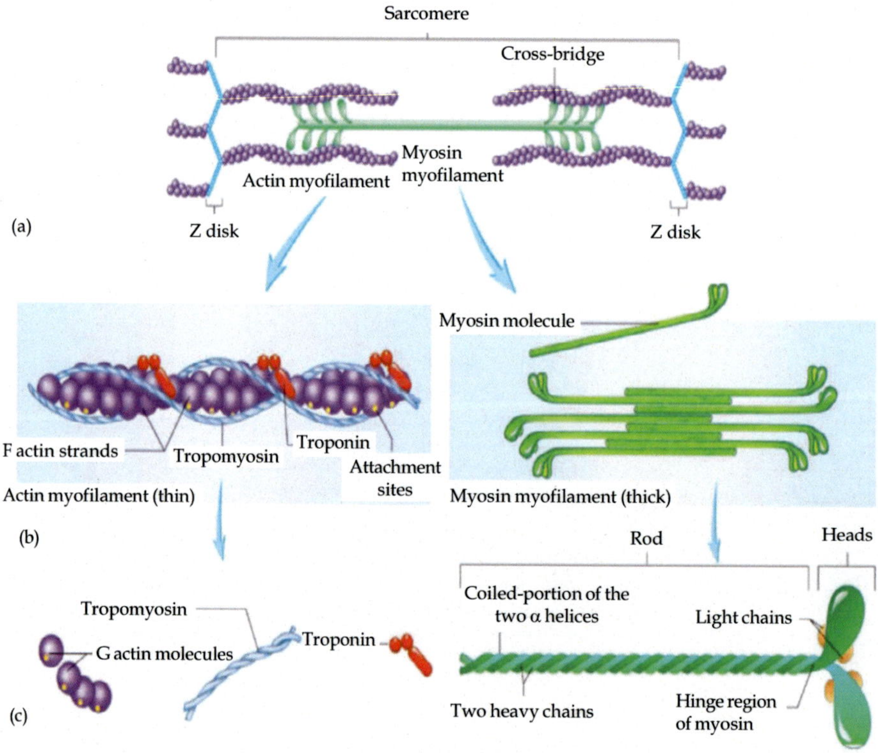

Myofilaments

Thick Filament

- Thick filaments are approximately 14 to 16 nm in diameter and 1.5 μM long.
- Thick filament constitute the A band of sarcomere.
- The thick filament contains 300-400 myosin molecules.

- The long tail of myosin consists of two polypeptides in a coiled helix terminating in two globular heads at one end.
- During muscle contractions each myosin head attaches to a G actin molecule of the actin filament.

Thin Filaments

- About 6 to 8 nm in diameter and they extended approximately 1.0 μm on either side of the Z disc.
- Thin filament or I band consist of two coiled strands of polymerized G-actin forming a double helix known as F-actin.
- F-actin combines with myosin to form the contractile actomyosin of active or pre-rigor muscle and the inextensible actomyosin of muscle in rigor mortis.

Z-Disk Ultra Structure

- Ultra thin filaments called Z filaments constitute the Z disk, and they connect with the actin filaments on either side of it.
- Near the Z disk, each actin filament connects to four Z filaments that pass obliquely through the Z disk.

Sarcoplasmic Reticulum and Transverse Tubules

- SR and T-tubules, with plasma membrane, conveys a neural impulse to the interior of each muscle cell and facilitates excitation-contraction coupling.
- The T-tubule system consists of a network of tubules which pass through the plasma membrane as tubular lumen.
- The T-tubule system terminates in the sarcoplasmic reticulum (SR) to which it is coupled at the SR-T tubule junction.
- The SR store, release, and sequesters intracellular calcium and also surrounds each myofibril.

Smooth Muscle

- Present in gastrointestinal tract, lungs and in uterus and vary in size and shape, depending on their location.
- The fibre shapes vary from extremely flattened to triangles and polyhedrons.

- The ratio of actin to myosin in smooth muscle is almost twice that of skeletal muscle.
- The smooth muscle fibre has a single nucleus usually centrally located within the cell.
- The sarcoplasmic reticulum is much less developed than skeletal muscle.

Cardiac Muscle

- Fibres of cardiac muscle are branched, main trunk larger in diameter than branches.
- Each fibre has a single centrally placed nucleus, the mitochondria are large and numerous.
- Myofilaments are not organized into myofibril, T-tubules are larger in diameter and located at the Z-disk.
- Fibres are held in place by connective tissue, intersected at regular intervals with intercalated disks.

Connective Tissue

- The connective tissue includes formed elements and amorphous ground substances.
- Connective tissue surrounding muscles, muscle bundles, and muscle fibres is fibrous and is known as connective tissue proper.
- Connective tissue proper consists of ground substance and extracellular fibres, collagen and elastin.
- Ground substance is a viscous solution containing soluble glycoproteins. *Hyaluronic acid* and *chondroitin sulfates* are the main glycoproteins in connective tissue.
- Extracellular fibres include *collagen, elastin* and *reticulin.*

❑❑❑

3

Composition and Nutritive Value of Meat

Composition of Muscle

Muscle tissue contains approximately 75% water and 25% solids, of which 19% are protiens. Lipids constitute about 2.5 to 5.0% of muscle.

1. Water

- This is the largest component comprising 65-75 of the muscle tissue. Due to polar behavior, water molecules are attached with electrically charged groups of muscle proteins.
- About 40% of the water is tightly bound and it is impossible to dislocate them.
- The attraction between protein and water molecules decreases as the distance increases. Thus most of the water remains in immobilized and free forms.
- When the pH of meat is more than isoelectric point, the negative charge of protein increases, results in retention of excess water.
- It may be noted that 70% of water of fresh meat is located in myofibrils. An increase WHC is associated with juiciness of cooked meat.

S.No.	Composition	Per cent (components)
1.	Water	75
2.	Protein	19
	a) Myofibrilar proteins	11.5 (Myosin, Actin, Tropomyosin, Toponin, Connectin)
	b) Sarcoplasmic proteins	5.5 (Myoglobin, Glycolytic enzymes)
	c) Connective tissue proteins	2.0 (Collagen, Elastin, Reticulin, Sarcolemma, S.R)
3.	Lipids	2.5
4.	Carbohydrates	1.2
5.	Misc. soluble substance	2.3 a) Nitrogenous substance- Creatine, IMP, Nucleotides.b) Inorganic-P, K, Na, Mg, Ca, Zn and trace element.
6.	Vitamins	Minute (Fat soluble, water soluble)

2. Protein

A) Myofibrillar protein

- Myofibrillar proteins contribute 95% of WHC and 75% of EC and to a large extent the tenderness
- These proteins make up about 60% of the total protein in muscle.
- Thick filament is composed of myosin protein. Length and diameter of thick filaments is 1.5µm and 14-16nm.

Contractile proteins: Proteins involved in muscle contraction

i) Myosin

- It is a long assyemetrical molecule containing a globular head and two identical polypeptides (tail). Myosin contributes 50-55% of myofibrillar proteins.
- It is the largest molecule biologically available with 1,800 $\bar{a}\,\bar{a}$. Tryptic digestion splits myosin into two large pieces- heavy and light meromyosin.
- The head portion carries the ATPase activity and have actin binding ability.

- This ATPase activity is stimulated by Ca++ and inhibited by Mg++ ion.
- Myosin and other proteins in thick filament are insoluble in water or dilute salt solution but are soluble in salt solutions of ionic strength 0.3-0.7.

ii) Actin

- The thin filament composed of mainly actin protein. Globular or G-actin is a monomer.
- At high ca++ ion strength and in presence of ATP, G-actin polymerized to fibrous protein F-actin.
- At low ionic strength F-actin depolymerizes to yield G-protein and contributes about 30-35% of myofibrilar protein.

Regulatory proteins: Proteins are associated with major myofibrillar proteins

i) Tropomyosin

- A fibrous protein occurs as a double helix, present in close association with thin filaments extending through the grooves of actin helix.

ii) Troponin

- Another regulatory protein present in thin filament cementing the tropomyosin thread into the grooves of actin at a regular interval.
- It is composed of three subunits.

  Tropomin-T: Binds tropomysin links to F-actin filaments.

  Troponin-C: Binds to calcium ions.

  Troponin-I: Inhibits interaction between actin-myosin in relaxed state.

iii) Actinin

- Alpha actinin, part of Z line and accelerate G-actin polymerisation. Beta actinin regulates the length of thin filaments.

Cytoskeletal proteins

- They maintain overall alignment and structural integrity of muscle and serve as the template for the sarcomere and myofilament.
- **'Gap filament'** is thin elastic filaments that form a bridge across the sarcomere and link two Z-discs.
- **Titin** is most abundant cytoskeletal protein, extends in each half of sarcomere from M-line to the Z-disk.

B) Sarcoplasmic proteins

- Soluble in water or dilute salt solutions, consist of glycolytic enzymes and myoglobin.
- It constitutes 2 percent of the skeletal muscle. Glycolytic proteins remained in bound form to the myofibliller proteins.

C) Stroma/connective tissue protein

Collagen

- It is the main fibrous protein in muscles and important determinant of tenderness.
- It makes up to 40-60% of the stroma protein and 20-25% of the total body protein.
- They are straight, inelastic and non brunching.
- At above 60°C these fibres transform to water soluble gelatin.
- The insoluble nature of collagen fibres is due to inter molecular cross linkages.
- These linkages increases with age and meat becomes tougher.

Elastin

- Less abundant than collagen, present in ligaments, arteries.
- Fibres are elastic, branched, do not hydrolyse by acids, alkali, enzyme and heat denaturation.
- It contains two unique amino acids desmin and isodesmin, cross links of them makes it so resistant.
- Can be hydrolysed by Ficin, Bromeline etc.

Reticulin

Composed of small fibres, intimate association with meristic acid. Forms network around blood vessels, nerves, epithelium etc. Function as intercellular cement.

Nutritive value of different species meat (raw)

Nutrients	Lamb	Pork	Beef	Chicken	Quail
Moisture (%)	71.50	71.95	71.60	74.86	71.50
Protein (%)	19.50	20.22	20.94	23.20	20.50
Fat (%)	7.00	6.75	6.33	3.50	5.50
Ash (%)	1.50	1.04	1.03	0.80	1.20
Calorie/ 100 g	145	147	147	125	125

3. Lipids

- Lipid is another major meat component. It is highly valuable and inversely proportional to the water content.
- Animal lipids are mainly neutral lipids and phospholipids. The neutral lipids are mostly triglycerides.
- The saturated and monounsaturated fatty acids predominate in meat lipids.
- The principal saturated fatty acids are palmitic and stearic acids, (C-16 and C-18).
- Most commonly occurring unsaturated fatty acids are oleic linoleic and linolenic acids.
- Phospholipids are present in small percentage (0.5-1%). They are mainly present in cell membranes.
- They may cause discolouration and off flavour in meat products.
- Cholesterol is a minor but important component of meat. Mostly it is in unesterifed form.

4. Carbohydrates

- Muscle normally contains very small amount of (1%) glycogen.
- However, it is fully exhausted before rigor mortis and important to achieve ultimate pH.

- They have important role in energy metabolism, glycolysis, influences the colour, tenderness and WHC.

5. Minerals

- About 3.5% of the total body weight is inorganic matter.
- Most of the inorganic matters are in skeleton as salt of calcium, phosphorus and magnesium.
- In the conversion of muscle to meat inorganic elements play an important role. Main function relates to development of rigor mortis, drop in pH, WHC.
- They also influence the colour and tenderization. Several inorganic ions act as catalysts for oxidative rancidity.

6. Vitamins

- The vitamin content of meat is variable depending on species, age, nutritional status and breed.
- Water soluble vitamins are localized in lean tissues, whereas, fat soluble vitamins in fatty tissues.
- Variety meats have substantial amounts of B-complex.
- Pork contains 5-10 times more thiamine as compared to mutton.
- Most of the vitamins in meat are relatively stable during processing or cooking.
- However, thiamine is to some extent susceptible to heat treatment.

4

Conversion of Muscle to Meat and Ageing

The muscle does not suddenly stop all living functions and become meat. Instead, a number of physical and chemical changes take place over a period of several hours or even days. This process is referred as the conversion of muscle to meat.

Homeostasis

- Maintenance of physiologically balanced internal environment controlled by nervous system and endocrine system.
- Homeostasis is lost within 4-6 minutes after bleeding.
- Many of the reaction in conversion due to homeostasis.
- Pre-slaughter conditions may alter post-mortem changes and affect meat quality.

Major Events

1. Exanguination
2. Circulatory failure
3. Post-mortem glycolysis and pH decline
4. Post-mortem heat production and dissipation
5. Rigor mortis–shortening and stiffness
6. Bacterial invasion
7. Loss of structural integrity
8. Enzymatic degradation

1. Exanguination

- The first step of slaughter, it marks beginning of post-mortem changes.

- Because of massive bleeding blood pressure gets decreased, heart pumping decrease and peripheral vessels constrict to maintain B.P.
- Maximum 50% of blood can be removed, rest remains in vital organs and muscles.

2. Circulatory failure

- Stopage of blood supply to muscles with the stoppage of heart
- Loss of oxygen supply, limited amount stored in myoglobin.
- Aerobic glycolysis by TCA cycle stops, leading to lack of energy supply for structural integrity.
- Depletion of ATP- ATPase produces inorganic phosphates, which stimulate anaerobic glycolysis.

3. PM glycolysis and pH decline

- In the absence of oxygen, anaerobic glycolysis leads to the formation of lactic acid from the glycogen reserves.
- The accumulation of lactic acid lowers muscle pH, an important post-mortem change.
- The rate and extent of pH decline varies with species, pre-slaughter factors, temperature, etc.
- The rate of pH decline is enhanced at high environmental temperature.
- A low ultimate pH is desired to check microbial growth.

A sharp decline in pH when the carcass is still hot may cause denaturation of proteins and the muscle look pale, soft and exudative (PSE).

Muscles with consistently high pH (due to depletion of glycogen before slaughter) during post-mortem changes look dark, firm and dry (DFD).

4. P. M. heat production and dissipation

- Because of circulatory failure, heat from deeper part of body not carried to lungs or surface for dissipation.
- Rise in muscle temperature–depends on metabolic rate and its duration, size and location of muscle, amount of fat cover.

- Scalding and singeing processes also influence heat dissipation.
- The temperature of slaughter hall and the duration of operation matters.

5. Rigor Mortis

- It refers to stiffening of muscle after death and one of the important phenomena during conversion of muscle to meat.
- The stiffening is due to formation of irreversible actomyosin crossbridges, since no energy is available to break the bond.
- Since the ATP level goes down, permanent actomyosin begins to form and gradually muscle becomes less extensible.
- Immediately after exsanguination, the actomyosin formation proceeds very slowly and the muscle is relatively extensible. This is called delay phase of rigor mortis.
- Then actomyosin forms faster and the muscle loose extensibility fast. This is called onset phase.
- When all the creatine phosphate is depleted, ADP can no longer be converted to ATP, muscle becomes quite stiff. This marks the completion of rigor mortis.

> **The apparent resolution of R.M is due to physical degradation of muscle structure in Z line area.**
>
> **Alkaline rigor- If the animal is exhausted before slaughter, rigor may develop even when the pH is high**

6. Bacterial invasion

- During post mortem period, body defence mechanisms stops, connective tissue cover fails, membrane properties altered and the muscle becomes susceptible to bacterial invasion.
- Due to failure of blood and lymphatic circulation, spread of microorganisms unavoidable.

7. Loss of structural integrity

- P.M. alteration of membrane properties initiates the degradation of muscular proteins. There will be progressive destruction of myofibrillar structure.

- The resolution of R.M. occurs due to disintegration in 'Z' line structure.
- A rapid decline in muscle pH causes denaturation of collagenous connective tissue.

8. Enzymatic Degradation

- Proteolytic enzymes called cathepsin hold in inactive state within lysosomes.
- As the pH declines these enzymes are released and begin to degrade the protein structure.
- The tenderization during P.M. ageing may be due to breakdown of some collagen by cathepsins.
- Early pH drop favours early release of cathepsin which also causes denaturation of proteins and degradation.

Changes in physical properties

a) *Colour:* normal muscle –bright red, P.M. muscle –dark purplish red, fresh muscle exposed – bright red

b) *Firmness:* Living muscle - tenacity - firm

R.M. muscle – very firm and stiff

After conversion –less firm

Severe denaturation –very soft

c) *WHC:* Proteins not denatured –high WHC -juicy and palatable;

pH of P.M. muscle very high – very high WHC

When pH drops –low WHC.

Ageing / Conditioning

- Holding of unprocessed meat above freezing point (-1.5) without microbial spoilage.
- When stored at 0-3^{0}C all the changes takes place in slow rate.
- The proteolytic enzymes are active, bring desirable changes, manifested by marked increase in flavor, juiciness and tenderness.

Changes during Ageing and Meat Quality

1. Protein denaturation

- This denaturation is due to higher temperature with low pH.
- At ultimate pH nearer to pI (5.4-5.5), most of the protein loses WHC and solubility.
- With rigor mortis muscle become tough, again it become soft and tender during ageing.
- This is due to detachment of actin filaments from 'Z' lines.
- At ultimate pH myoglobin converted to metmyoglobin (discolouration).
- During ageing meat pH tends to increase.

2. Proteolysis

- Denaturation of protein facilitates proteolysis.
- This is initiated by the release of CASF which causes 'Z' line disintegration by degrading desmin, connectin, nebulin, troponin, tropomyosin.
- CASF act above pH-6, cathepsins acts below pH 5 can degrade actin and myosin, collagen.
- Collagen fibres appear to swell and cross links are broken, but they are not denatured or hydrolysed.
- Resolution of rigor is loss of structural integrity by enzymatic degradation.

3. Other chemical changes

- ATP → ADP → IMP → Inosinic acid → hypoxanthine (flavor component).
- The rate is higher at high pH and temperature (0°C →10 to 13 day, 30°C → 10 to 13 hours).
- Breakdown of protein and fat during conditioning also contributes to flavour.

❑❑❑

5

Meat Quality and Spoilage

Physico-Chemical Quality of Meat

Some characteristics of fresh and raw meat need to be properly understood in order to achieve the best in processing :

- Meat which has undergone post-mortem changes after slaughter but has not been subjected to any processing is called fresh meat.
- Meat which has undergone freezing can be termed as meat.

1. Meat colour

- Visual perception of meat on hue, chroma and value
- Hue – primary colour; chroma- intensity; value – brightness.
- Meat colour depends on quality and chemical state of myoglobin.
- Colour of meat varies between species, sex, age, muscles.
- Myoglobin constitutes 80-90% of total meat pigments.
- Myoglobin content of more active species and muscle is higher.

Colour of meat and myoglobin % in various species

Species	Meat colour	Myoglobin (%)
Chicken	Grey white-dull red	0.02
Sheep/goat	Light to dark red	0.06
Pig	Gryaish pink	0.25
Cattle/Buffalos	Cherry red	0.50

Characteristics of myoglobin (Mg)

- In intact meat iron in heme remains in reduced form.
- On exposure to air it forms oxy-myoglobin which gives bright red colour (desirable).
- Normally oxymyoglobin is stable and not easily oxidized.
- In less oxygen, Mg or oxy-Mg is oxidized to brown colour metmyoglobin.
- To prevent this, fresh meat should be packed in oxygen permeable films.
- Keeping near freezing point advised for maintaining colour.

2. Water holding capacity

- The capacity of meat to retain its water against physical forces.
- This contributes to the juiciness and influences tenderness and colour also.
- Fresh meat with good WHC has less shrinkage during cooking.
- Water exists in three different forms- free water, immobilized water and bound water.
- Those hold by capillary forces on the surface are free water, can be removed by minor physical force.
- The middle layer remains in contact with proteins are immobilized water, can be removed by strong physical forces.
- However 4-5% of water tightly bound to charged groups of proteins, cannot be removed by any physical force.
- At ultimate pH the WHC is minimum; it is called net charge effect.
- Changes associated with rigor mortis also reduce WHC, called steric effect.

3. Marbling

- It refers to the intramuscular fat which can be visibly detected in cut surface of muscle.

- The solidification of fat during chilling contributes to firmness of meat.
- Marbling is important parameter in USDA grading system.
- Some specified cuts like chops and steaks retain uniform thickness and typical shape due to marbling.
- Moderately marbled meat yield juicy and flavourful taste.
- Too little marbling yield dry and flavourless. Excess marbling not desired.

4. Connective tissue

- Amount of connective tissue is directly related to texture characteristics, more active muscles deposit more connective tissue to gain strength.
- This leads to coarse texture of biceps femoris and tenderness of loin muscle.
- In fact it increases the muscle fibre diameter and fibre bundles which leads to tough texture of meat.

5. Firmness

- This is an important parameter for carcass setting, fabrication, ageing, processing, slicing etc.
- During chilling firmness increases due to loss of extensibility.
- Fresh meat with high WHC shows firmness and tight structure.
- Meat with good degree of firmness yields better processed product.

Microbial Quality

- Meat is a highly perishable food item. Hence, utmost precautions must be taken to safeguard it right from bleeding of slaughter animals till final consumption.
- Meat gets contaminated during slaughter and dressing operations.
- These organisms proliferate and cause deteriorative changes in meat unless proper measures are taken to retard their growth.

Sources of microbial contamination

- Hides/skin and feet.
- Gastrointestinal contaminants
- Instruments such as knives, cleavers, saws, hooks etc.
- Water used for washing carcasses and instruments
- Airborne contamination
- Hands and clothing of the personnel

Types of microorganism

- The microorganisms that occur in meat may be bacteria or fungi.
- Fungi may be multi-cellular filaments (molds) or large single cells with buds (yeast).
- Molds are capable of producing minute spores under unfavourable conditions.
- Fungi gain upper hand over bacteria in meat when it is semi-dry.
- Bacterial growth or multiplication takes place in phases.

Factors affecting growth of microorganism

Intrinsic factors

1. *Water activity:* The amount of water available in a food system for the growth of microorganism is generally expressed in terms of water activity (a_w).
    - Fresh meat generally has a_w of 0.99 or more.
    - Most meat spoilage bacteria can grow only up to a_w of 0.91 but most spoilage mold and yeast can grow up to a a_w of 0.86.
2. *pH:* Meat pH is yet another intrinsic factor which influences the growth of microorganisms.
    - Bacterial growth is best at neutral pH.
    - When ultimate pH (5.5) is reached, bacterial growth is reduced to a large extent and the growth of mold and yeast is favoured.

3. *Redox potential:* Redox potential refers to the reducing or oxidizing conditions prevailing on meat and this factor also influences the growth of microorganisms.
4. *Nutrient content:* Presence of protein, fat, carbohydrates, vitamins etc. in meat.

Extrinsic factors

1. *Temperature:* All microorganisms has an optimum temperature for growth.
   - Optimum temperature for psychrophiles below 20°C, thermophiles above 45°C and mesophiles between 20-45°C.
   - A refrigerated temperature of nearly 5°C greatly retards the growth of most psychrophilic organisms responsible for the spoilage of meat.
   - These bacteria generally belong to genera *Pseudomonas, Achromobactor, Flavobacterium, Micrococcus, Streptococcus,* in fresh meat and *Lactobacillus* in cured or vacuum packed meat.
2. *Oxygen:* Availability of oxygen determines the type of microbes for growth.
   - Bacteria found in meat may be either aerobic or anaerobic or sometimes facultative.
   - Bacteria that grow on the surface of fresh meat are generally aerobes,
   - All molds and yeast that grow in meat are aerobic in nature.
3. *Relative humidity:* It is the amount of moisture available around the food.
   - Meat undergoes surface spoilage from molds, yeasts and certain bacteria at high R.H.
   - Improperly wrapped meats suffer surface spoilage in the refrigerator due to high R.H.
4. *Gases:* Presence of oxygen around the meat determine the type of microbes to grow.
   - The storage of food in normal atmosphere undergoes aerobic spoilage.
   - Increased amount of CO_2 and ozone (O_3) are effective in retarding surface spoilage.

Spoilage of Meat

- When total bacterial population is above 10^7/g most signs of spoilage appears on meat.
- Under aerobic conditions, significant sign of meat spoilage by bacteria and yeast is the slime formation on the surface.
- There may be discoloration of meat due to oxidizing agents produced by bacteria.
- Production of off-odours is also common.
- Bacterial action causes proteolysis of meat proteins and lipolysis of meat lipids. Residual carbohydrates yield skatol and indole.
- Molds may grow on semi-dried meats causing surface stickiness and whiskers.
- Under anaerobic conditions, meat decomposition is more offensive.
- There may be putrefaction in the deep tissues and bone joints, which is accompanied by foul odours or taints.
- Souring may also develop due to accumulation of organic acids.
- Canned meats may suffer chemical or biological spoilage or both.

Aerobic spoilage

Spoilage by bacteria- surface slime- by Pseudomonas, Acenetobacter, Alcaligens, Streptococcus, Leuconostoc, Micrococcous.

- Lactobacillus and Leuconostoc cause the greening of sausages.
- Oxidation of fat produces tallowy flavour, whereas, hydrolysis gives rise to rancid flavour.
- Rancidity also caused by lipolytic bacteria namely Pseudomonas and Achromobacter.
- Various types of off odours or tastes due to spoilage of meat.

Various surface colour due to pigmented bacteria :	
Serratia marcescens	Red spot
Pseudomonas syncyanea	Blue colour
Micrococcus, Flavobacterium	Yellow
Chromobacterium	Greenish blue or Brownish black

Spoilage by yeast: Causing sliminess, lipolysis, off-odours and tastes, and discolouration-white, cream, pink, or brown.

Spoilage by molds: Stickiness due to incipient growth of molds, decomposition of fat due to hydrolysis by lipases, off-odours and tastes giving a musty flavour and colour changes.

- Whiskers- Thamnidium, Mucor, Rhizopus
- Black spot- *Cladosporium herbarum*
- White spot- *Sporotrichum carnis*
- Green patches-*Penicillium* spp.

Anaerobic spoilage

Anaerobic bacteria can grow in meat under anaerobic conditions and cause spoilage.

- *Souring:* Sour odour and taste caused by fatty acids-formic, acetic, butyric, propionic or organic acids- lactic and succinic.
- *Putrefaction:* decomposition of protein with production of foul smelling compounds- H_2S, mercaptans, indole, skatol, ammonia, and amines. Usually caused by Clostridium, Pseudomonas, Alkaligenes and Proteus.
- *Taint:* off odour and taste by souring or putrefaction next to the bones, especially in hams, predominantly caused by *Enterococci.*

❑❑❑

6

Meat Preservation by Chilling and Freezing

Why Preservation

- Meat is a highly perishable commodity due to nearly neutral pH, high moisture content and rich nutrients.
- Contamination with spoilage organisms is almost unavoidable which makes meat most susceptible to spoilage.
- Unless proper preservation methods are adopted, deteriorative microbial activity, enzymatic and chemical reactions along with physical changes are bound to occur.
- Once meat is contaminated with microorganisms, their removal is difficult; hence preservation of meat is very important.

What is Preservation

- Preservation prevents the spoilage of food by means of preventing the activity of microorganisms.
- Preservation of meat is usually accomplished by the use of low temperature, high temperature, moisture control, direct microbial inhibition etc.
- To retain the wholesomeness, nutritive value and quality of meat by controlling the growth of micro-organisms.
- To minimize or arrest chemical, physical and physiological changes of an undesirable nature.

Principles of Food Preservation

1. Prevention or delay of microbial decomposition.
2. Prevention or delay of self decomposition.
3. Prevention of damage due to insects, physical causes.

Methods of preservation

Meat Preservation			
↓	↓	↓	↓
Controlling Temp	Moisture control	Chemical preservative	Other treatment
↓	↓	↓	↓
1. Lowering Temperature	1. Dehydration	1. Curing	1. Irradiation
a) Chilling/ refrigeration	a) Drying	2. Smoking	2. High pressure
b) Freezing	b) Freeze drying	3. Antibiotics	3. Packaging
2. Increasing Temperature	2. IMM	4. Antioxi- dants	4. Edible coating
a) Pasteurization	3. Fermentation		
(broiling, frying, steaming etc)			
b) Sterilization (canning, retorting)			

Preservation by Low Temperature

- Low temperature is used to retard the chemical or enzyme reactions and to slow down or stop growth and activity of micro organisms in food.
- The most common method of preservation of meat by low temperature is refrigeration (-2 to 5°c) and freezing (-18^{0}C).
- Refrigeration slow the microbial growth rate however freezing prevents the growth of almost all food borne micro organisms.

Chilling

- Chilling is the storage above freezing point usually by ice or by mechanical refrigeration.
- Refrigeration is done by use of refrigerants like ammonia, ethylene chloride or freon gas
- The most common method of prolonging of shelf life of meat is by chilling.
- Refrigeration is single most important means of preservation of fresh meat.

- The preservative action of refrigeration is based on the prevention and multiplication of harmful bacteria.
- The modern meat industry is based on efficient refrigeration.
- Chilling is fundamental operation for applying cold to the meat to reduce its temperature quickly.

Mode of chilling

- Cooling of carcasses is done by using cold water, air, solid CO_2, liquid N_2 etc.
- Most common medium in practice is ice-water or chilled air.
- Rapid cooling occurs when the medium is very cold and the meat surfaces are in continuous contact.
- Immersion chilling of poultry in cold water or in slush ice widely used.
- A combination of immersion chilling and air blast cooling is also used.

Quick chilling is better: saving time and space; better keeping quality; shrinkage of meat reduced; bloom is enhanced.

Factors affecting chilling rate

i) Size of the carcass/pack
ii) Covering of subcutaneous fat
iii) Initial temperature of the meat/product
iv) Temperature of the medium
v) Circulation of air over the carcass.

Methods of chilling

1. **Immersion Chilling:** The carcasses are immersed in cold water for an extended period of time. It may be still water chilling and mechanically agitated water chilling. The later may have water with counter or co-current flow. Immersion chilling of poultry may take for 1-12 hrs depending upon size, weight, temperature.
2. **Spray Chilling:** It is an alternative to immersion chilling. Spraying of cold water is used. High amount of water required, uneconomical and ecologically unacceptable.

3. **Air Chilling:** Birds hung in rack which is pushed into rooms at 0°C. Cold air is blown gently over the carcasses. It may take 40 min to 12hrs.
4. **Cryogenic Chilling:** Liquid N_2 or CO_2 used as cooling agent. These are more commonly used for freezing.

Storage life

- Depends on initial microbial load, temperature, relative humidity, covering, species and type of product.
- Normally it is 3 days, maximum 4 days under ideal condition.
- Pork, poultry, fish spoils faster due to oxidation.

Chilling of poultry carcass

- Poultry should be chilled rapidly at the earliest after evisceration.
- Commercially by ice water with continuous agitation of carcass for quick chilling.
- Poultry chilling is completed within 2 hr in ice chilling.
- Air temperature of 0°C, air speed from 0.75-1.5 m/sec and R.H. 90-95% is desirable.

Cold shortening

- When pre-rigor meat is fast chilled below 15°C, there is shortening of muscles.
- This shortening or contraction is more at 0°C and still more at -2°C.
- A 40% shortening is quite common, meat becomes very tough.
- When shortening exceeds 40%, Z-lines are disrupted and meat becomes tender.
- Cold shortening can be avoided by keeping the meat above 14°C till the rigor stage.

Freezing

Storage of meat below freezing point is called freezing. It is an excellent method for preservation of meat. Freezing helps in maintaining the quality of meat/products for long time by minimizing physical, biochemical and microbial changes. Freezing retains the original quality attributes of meat to a great extent.

Changes during freezing

- Chemical and enzymatic reactions slows down,
- Formation of ice crystals, expansion in volume, water drawn out from cells.
- Increase concentration of solutes in cells hastens salting out, dehydration, denaturation of proteins.
- Meat becomes irreversibly dehydrated.

Effect of freezing on microbes

i) Very low temperature retards/stops most enzyme and bacterial activity

ii) Water in ice form is not available for bacterial growth and multiplication.

iii) Complete immobilization, reduces spreading of organisms by convection.

iv) Microorganisms cannot grow and slowly die.

v) Lethal effects due to denaturation of proteins/enzymes and by cold shock.

Slow freezing

- A continuous freezing boundary forms and slowly proceeds inwards.
- Temperature remains near freezing point for a long time.
- Temperature employed -15 to -30°C, time taken to freeze 3-72hrs.
- Large extracellular ice crystals forms.
- More loss through drip during thawing.

Fast freezing

- Frozen at below -30°C in short time (within 30 min).

- Immersion, indirect contact or by air blast freezing.
- Numerous small ice crystals form, both intra and extra cellularly.
- Small ice crystal causes less damage, less drip loss during thawing.

Advantages of fast freezing

1. Small ice crystals, less mechanical damage.
2. Less time for diffusion of solutes.
3. Prompt prevention of microbial growth.
4. Rapid reduction of enzyme activity.
5. Thermal shock to micro organism.

Freezing Methods

1. Still air

Air is the medium of heat transfer, meat freezes very slowly. Temperature -10 to -30°C used. Large quantity should not be kept. Heat loss by convection.

2. Plate freezer

Medium is metal. Flat surfaces of meat packets are directly placed on freezer plates. Temperature ranges -10 to -30°C. Thin packets are more suitable. Conduction is the process of heat loss, slightly faster, can be speeded up by cold air circulation.

3. Blast freezing

Most commonly used commercially. Cold air is blasted with rapid circulation. Rate of heat transfer increased by air movement. Freezing rate faster, also called fast frozen. Temperature -10 to -40°C.

4. Liquid immersion / liquid sprays

Most common for poultry. Higher rates of heat transfer, so higher temperature are used, freezing rate comparable. The liquid should be non toxic, high conductivity, low viscosity and freezing point.

5. Cryogenic freezing

Three systems may be used- direct immersion, spray liquid or vapour circulation. The common agents are nitrogen either vapour of liquid. Carbon dioxide liquid or solid, sometimes liquid N_2O is used.

Frozen Storage

- The frozen meat is transferred to the frozen chamber where the temperature, RH and air circulation should be adequate.
- The manner in which frozen meat is stored influences the quality than the process of freezing itself.
- As a rule storage temperature is around (-18°C to -25°C) and R.H is (92-95%).
- The storage life is 6-12 months depending upon initial quality of the product.
- Repeated freezing not recommended, never refreeze a product as a last resort to save it.

Storage life of meat & meat products in freezer at-18°C

Item	Months
Beef	12
Ground Beef	10
Pork	6
Ground pork	6
Veal	9
Lamb	9
Chicken	12
Fish	12
Offal (edible)	24
Sausage	4

Thawing

- Process of warming the frozen meat to melt the ice inside.
- Thawing occurs more slowly than freezing.
- Rate of thawing depends on product temperature, size, medium and its temperature.

- Thawing causes greater damage to meat than freezing.
- Thawing of meat should be done with package preferably in refrigerator.
- Frozen meat may be thawed quickly by keeping in running water.
- Drip is proportional to rate of thawing.

Drip- The pink or reddish liquid comes out after thawing.

Thawing of meat can be done by: Refrigerator > normal atmosphere > in normal water > hot water > direct cooking > microwave oven, (in ascending order of rate).

Problems during freezing

Freezer burn: This is characterized by a browning or light color such as chicken skin. It results from the loss of moisture at the surface, leaving the product more porous. This is irreversible; affect both raw and cooked meat. It is due to improper packaging. It appears dry, grainy and brownish.

Thaw Rigor: When pre-rigor meat is frozen, a severe type of rigor mortis ensues during thawing. The shortening may be 60 to 80% of the original length of the muscle. The condition results in tough meat and heavy drip losses.

Bone darkening: A condition induced by freezing and thawing of young chicken. The red color is due to haemoglobin causing dark discolouration, commonly occur around leg, thigh and knee joint. It does not affect the flavour or texture, pre cooling can solve the problem.

Oxidation: Oxidation during frozen storage continues very slowly, especially to the processed meat products. Salt acts as a catalyst in oxidation reaction.

❑❑❑

7

Meat Preservation by Canning, Drying and Irradiation

High Temperature Preservation

Preservation of meat by using high temperature is based on their destructive effects on microorganism and to inactivate some endogenous enzymes that could cause deteriorative changes. In meat preservation, there are two temperature categories in common use-pasteurization and sterilization.

a) Pasteurization

The term pasteurization implies moderate heating, during which product reach temperatures of 58 to 75°C, is employed in cooking most processed meat. Shelf life of meat products is extended by pasteurization, but they must be stored under refrigeration.

b) Sterilization

Sterilization means the destruction of all viable organisms including spores of most resistance *Cl. botulinum*. Canned meat are sometimes called commercially sterile to indicate that no viable organisms can be detected by the usual cultural methods employed or that number of survivors is so low as to be of no significance under the conditions of canning and storage.

Factors affecting heat resistance of microorganisms in meat

1. *Moisture content:* Heat resistance decrease with increase in H_2O content.
2. *Fat content:* In general increase heat resistance with the increase in fat content in meat as it has some protective effect on microbes.

3. *Salt level:* Use of salt in meat products reduces a_w, thereby increase heat resistance.
4. *Sugar level:* Addition of sugar in the products also increases of heat resistance in similar manner to that of the salt.
5. *pH:* Microbes are more heat resistant at neutral pH.
6. *Proteins:* Have some protective effect thereby increase heat resistance.
7. *Number of organisms:* Larger the number of microbes, higher the degree of heat resistance.
8. *Inhibitory compounds*: Heat resistance of most microbes reduces in the presence of heat resistant antibiotics, SO_2, nitrite etc.

Adverse changes induced by heat

1. Protein denaturation which results in shrinkage and loss of fluid.
2. Accelerate oxidative rancidity.
3. Maillard reaction products cause burnt flavour.
4. Warmed over flavour (WOF) when cooked products are packed hot or reheated after storage.

Canning of Meat

- "Canning is a process by which food products are thermo-processed in hermetically sealed container" - Nicolas Appert is the pioneer.
- Canning provides meat with desirable quality and long storage life.
- In canning, meats are subjected to heat treatment to kill spoilage microorganisms.
- The heat treatment is given after packing in cans or in retort pouches.
- Pasteurization- internal temperature 65 to 75°C, cans stored at refrigerator.
- Commercial sterilization- internal temperature of 121°C, sufficient to kill all spores, stored at room temperature.

- Pasteurized canned meat has a shelf life upto 2 years at refrigerator.
- Sterilized can have a shelf life up to two years at ambient temperature and 4-5 years at refrigeration.

Can material: Low carbon steel plate coated with tin is commonly used. To prevent interaction between meat and metals sulfur resistant internal lacquer (oleoresins, epoxy resins or epoxyphenolics) are used.

Retort

- A retort is a steel tank in which cans are heat processed.
- Retorts are pressure vessels operate in high pressure using steam or superheated water.
- There are three types of retort - non-agitating, continuous agitating and hydrostatic.
- Non-agitating retort is loaded, closed and processed as a batch
- Hydrostatic retort is space saving, low operating cost and greater capacity but require large initial investment.

Canning procedure

1. *Preparation and filling*: Inedible parts like bones, cartilages, tendons and excess fat are removed from meats, then preheated and placed in cans.
2. *Exhausting and sealing*: After filling the cans are exhausted by heating or vacuum, then hermetically sealed. Exhausting prevents expansion of contents, reduce oxygen level and chemical reaction.
3. *Thermal processing*: After sealing the cans are subjected to heating either by low temperature (65-70°C) or high temperature (>100°C).
4. *Cooling*: After processing cans should be cooled promptly to prevent undue changes in texture and colour of the product.
5. *Can washing*: Then the cans are washed thoroughly with potable water to remove dust and grease.
6. *Outside lacquering*: A coloured varnish containing vegetable resin or synthethic resin is applied outside to prevent rusting of cans.

Aseptic canning

In this process meat products and cans are sterilized separately then filled into sterilized cans under sterile atmosphere. But it is difficult to maintain sterile conditions during filling and sealing of cans.

Retort pouch processing

- Multiple layer (laminates) flexible pouches are used instead of metal cans.
- Product is filled in these pouches and subjected to high temperature process.
- As these are made up of thin layers, heating and cooling is very rapid.
- The quality of products is better maintained and easy to open a pouch than a can.

Common defect in can

Buckling: This happens due to improper exhaustion of air in the can.

Paneling: It occurs due to over exhaustion of can during sealing.

Flipper: One end becomes convex by striking with a hard object or heating due to gas production.

Springer: Springer is can with both the end bulged. If one end is pushed, the other pops out due to gas production.

Soft swell: Can has both ends bulged but may be dented by pressing.

Hard swell: Cannot be dented by hands. These are often hydrogen swells by the action of acid on iron.

Preservation of Meat by Moisture Control

- Dried or low moisture foods are those contain less than 25% moisture with a water activity (a_w) below 0.60.
- Freeze dried meat also comes under this category.
- Shelf stable foods should have moisture between 15-50% with an a_w of 0.60 to 0.85.

- Meat usually cooked before dehydration.
- The final moisture content after drying should be approximately 4% for beef and pork.

1. Dehydration / Drying

Removal of water available for microbial growth in the meat. The extent of availability of water to microbial cell is expressed by water activity (a_{-w}). Dehydration lowers the water activity considerably to prevent the growth of spoilage organisms.

Sun drying

- Direct sun light for drying of meat is the oldest technique for preservation of meat.
- The products are generally contaminated with dust particles etc.
- Not good for dehydration and rehydration.

Mechanical drying

- Drying process with hot air oven and controlled humidity,
- Sometime cabinet dryer is used for large scale drying.
- Such meat has difficulty in dehydration and rehydration.
- Often a dried thick layer is formed on the surface, called case hardening.

Pemmican: Sun dried meat pounded and then covered with melted fat and fruits (North American Indian).

Charqui/Jerki: Muscle strip light salted followed by air drying (South America). This is also known as Biltong in South Africa.

Beef jerky is a cured and smoked, restructured product. It is thinly sliced, marinated dried product that does not require refrigeration.

Physical aspects of drying

- The size of the meat has an effect on the time of drying.
- Heat damage is characterized by toughness, grittiness, burnt flavor.

- High fat content- slow rate of drying.
- A low grade meat is preferred for drying.
- In overcooked meat connective tissue changed to gelatin, reconstitute quickly,
- Undercooked meat, slow drying and reconstitution.

Organoleptic aspects of dried meat

- Long term storage of dried meat must be in airtight and moisture proof container.
- Airtight package will maintain flavor of dried meat for 12 months at 15^0C.
- Dried meat stored in presence of oxygen at high temperature become pale to yellow.
- Precooking the meat before drying greatly reduces its lipolytic activity.
- Rancidity may also be avoided by gas packing the dehydrated meat.
- Dried meat with above 10% moisture, mould growth may occur after some weeks

Freeze drying of meat

- Freeze drying involves the removal of water from meat by sublimation from the frozen state to vapour state by keeping it under vacuum and low heat treatment.
- It has better rehydration ability, nutritive quality and acceptability.
- The major use of freeze dried meats is in dehydrated soup mixes.
- Meat with low fat is used to minimize rancidity problem.

Freeze drying process

- In freeze drying, actual freezing is preceded by the precooking of meat.
- Meat is first frozen at -40°C then dried under vacuum at low temperature in plate heat exchanger.

- Ice crystals get sublimated to water vapour and there is no rise in temperature.
- In first phase free and immobilized water (90-95%) is removed.
- In second phase remaining water is removed at higher temperature.
- Freeze dried meats are packed in vacuum for longer storage stability.

Accelerated freeze drying (AFD)

In this case heat is given to the plate preferably at 60^0C to enhance heat exchange during the initial phase of sublimation and to supply heat for drying during the second phase.

Stability of freeze dried meat depends on

- Method of drying.
- Residual moisture content.
- Packaging technique.
- Storage condition.
- Quality of raw material.

Advantages of freeze drying

- Retain original shape and size.
- Very porous (honey comb appearance).
- Readily rehydrable, resembles fresh meat.
- No case hardening, minimum moisture, resists spoilage.
- No denaturation of protein, biological properties retained.
- Light weight, better palatability and nutritive value.

2. Intermediate moisture meat (IMM)

Prepared by hurdle concept-combination of reduced pH, a_w, certain additives such as glycerol, glycol, sorbitol, sucrose etc as humectants, certain fungistats such as sorbate and benzoate.

- These are shelf stable meat products, having moisture content of 15-50% and a_w between 0.50 to 0.85.
- In preparing IMM, water may be removed by adsorption, desorption
- In adsorption, meat first freeze dried then by controlled humidification desired composition achieved.
- In desorption, meat placed in a solution of higher osmotic pressure at equilibrium, the desired a_w is reached.

Irradiation

Electromagnetic radiations are continuous waves capable of ionising molecules in their path.

Electromagnetic radiation is known to inhibit the growth of microorganisms.

Cold sterilization - microbial destruction of meat takes place without significantly raising the temperature in meat.

U.V. Rays

- Maximum effect at 2500 A^0 produced by mercury vapour lamps.
- Have bactericidal effect, no penetration power
- Spores & moulds are resistant, yeast more resistant.
- Suitable for surface sterilization.
- Used in ageing of meat to control the growth of surface organisms.

Ionizing radiation

- Electro-magnetic radiation of short wavelength and high energy in the form of x rays.
- Among the alpha, beta and gama rays, only gama rays have penetration power (30cm).
- Gamma rays produced by breakdown of radioactive elements (^{60}Co,^{137}Cs).
- Ionizing radiation destroys microorganisms by affecting DNA & RNA.

- Temperature raised is very less (only 2°C) and called as cold sterilization.
- Affect taste and odour above 5 kGy by forming volatile sulphur containing substances.
- Beef is more affected compared to pork.
- Flavor damage can be reduced by freezing meat, adding vitamin C.
- It cannot inactivate enzymes which cause problem in long storage.

Uses

- Decontamination of carcasses.
- Reducing the pathogens such as *Salmonella, Campylobacter* and *Listeria* in meat and meat products.
- Extension of shelf-life of meat and meat products.
- Irradiating poultry carcasses with 2.5 kGy eliminate *Salmonella* and extend shelf life by 2 times at 5°C.
- A dose of 50-100 Krad can enhance shelf life of fresh meat cuts and sterilize pork, poultry and fish.
- Radurisation- low dose (0.75 to 2.5 kGy) irradiation intended to increase the shelf life of food. By this meat can be stored for 5 weeks at 3°C.
- Radicidation (pasteurization) 2.5–10 kGy increase shelf life without adverse effect.
- Used to destroy the specific organism, E.g. *Taenia solium* in meat with 1 kGy.
- Radappertization (cold sterilization)- this is high dose irradiation, 30-40 kGy is used. This will completely destroy all microorganisms and sterilise the meat completely. Meat is first cooled to -196°C by liquid nitrogen then subjected to radiation.

8

Meat Preservation by Curing, Smoking and Chemicals

Curing

Curing actually means salting, used for fish preservation 3500 BC. Modern meat curing started 1950 onwards, salt along with sugar etc are injected for preservation, color and flavor. Traditionally curing of meat is limited to pork (ham & belly) and beef (brisket & leg muscles).

Major curing ingredients

Salt

- Basic for all curing mixtures, it acts by dehydration and altering the osmotic pressure thus prevents bacterial growth and spoilage of meat.
- Chloride ions in the salt directly act on microorganisms.
- It slows down the action of proteolytic enzymes in meat.
- It gives a hard and dry product with dark color when salt alone is added.
- Commonly 65 degree brine used, in ham -3% bacon- 2%

Sugar

- Mainly used to improve flavour by moderating the action of salt.
- Counteract the harsh hardening effects of salt by less drying' enhance flavour and colour through browning reaction.
- Acts as preservative by retarding bacterial growth.
- Generally used up to 1-2%, corn syrup can be used in place of sugar.

Nitrates/nitrites

- Imparts colour, flavour, antibacterial and antioxidant.
- Mainly used for *Clostridium botulinum.*
- Leads to the formation of nitrosamines which is carcinogenic,
- *Perigo factor-* anti bacterial property increased after heating with nitrates.

Phosphates (alkaline)

- Increase water binding and yield by raising pH and unfolding of proteins.
- Prevents rancidity by chelating metal ions.

Ascorbates/erythorbates

- Enhance and stabilize colour.
- Reduce MMb to Mb and accelerates curing reaction, increases yield of NO from HNO_3.
- Acts as antioxidant and stabilize colour.
- Reduce nitrosamine formation.

Curing reaction

$$\text{Nitrate} \xrightarrow{\text{Nitrate reducing organisms}} \text{Nitrite}$$

$$\text{Nitrite} \xrightarrow{\text{Absence of light and air}} \text{Nitric oxide (NO)}$$

$$\text{NO} + \text{Mb} \longrightarrow \text{Nitric oxide metmyoglobin (NOMMb)}$$

$$\text{NOMMb} \xrightarrow{\text{Favourable conditions}} \text{Nitric oxide myoglobin (NOMb) (unstable cured pigment)}$$

$$\text{NOMb + heat/smoke} \longrightarrow \text{Nitroso haemochromogen (stable pink pigment)}$$

Curing Methods

1. Dry curing

- Here salt, sugar and nitrite/nitrate is used for country ham or bacon.

- It is good for fatty cuts, nitrite should be used for better colour.
- High cost due to poor space used, high inventory by slow curing, harsh salty flavour.

2. Pickle curing

- Curing ingredients dissolved in water to make pickle or brine.
- Strength of brine 60-70 degree, time required almost same as dry curing.
- Poor space utilization, slow turnover of inventories.

3. Artery pumping

- Pumping of pickle through arterial system (8-10% of weight).
- Mainly limited for hams and picnics.
- Needles inserted into the femoral artery, through which pickle goes to entire ham
- Fast curing, rapid turnover, high yield, improved by phosphates.
- Only hams and picnics are useful, care required having intact artery.

4. Injection curing

- Single or multiple needles with multiple holes are used.
- About 10% w/w pickle 65 degrees injected.
- It leads to cure accumulation, needs longer time for diffusion.
- Yields more, reduce production cost, quality not as good as dry cured bacon.

5. Hot curing

- Hot pickles are applied by artery/stitch pumping.
- Rapid curing and faster processing and turnover of inventory.
- Yield higher than dry curing lesser than injection.
- No pickle pockets, improved flavour.
- Problem in heating and applying curing,

Curing ingredients, their maximum permissible limits (MPL) and functions

Ingredient	MPL / Limit	Functions
Sodium chloride	1.5 – 5.0 %	Cured meat flavour
Cane sugar	1.0 – 1.5 %	flavour
Sodium nitrite	200 ppm	Colour & flavour
Sodium nitrate	500 ppm	antibotulimum
Alkaline phosphate	0.5 %	Improve WHC, texture, juiciness, emulsification, antioxidant, antimicrobial

Smoking

Nomadic man discovered preservative effect and desirable flavour in meat hung near fire (due to smoke). Smoking practiced from when recorded history begins.

In modern days smoking serves the variety flavour, because preservation is not a problem.

Purposes

1. Development of flavour
2. Preservation
3. Creation of new products
4. Develop colour
5. Protection from oxidation
    - Smoking and cooking together develops colour of cured meat due to Maillard reaction which gives brown colour on the surface.
    - Smoking extends the shelf life because of its antibacterial and antioxidant properties.
    - Phenols and acids contribute bacteriostatic and bactericidal effect.

Production of smoke

- Hard wood (40-60% cellulose, 20-30% hemi-cellulose, 20-30% lignin) used for smoking.

- Burning at 650-750^{0}Fàbest quality smoke produced, but above 700^{0}F (370^{0}C), polycyclic hydrocarbons (PCHs, carcinogenic) are produced.
- To minimize PCH burning at 650^{0}F (350 ^{0}C) is better.

Composition and action of smoke

Major components of wood smoke are phenols, alcohols, carbonyls, hydrocarbons, and gases of which phenols, aldehyde and carbonyls are most important.

- Phenols have 3 properties-Antioxidant, colour & flavour and bacteriostatic
- Antioxidant property of smoke mainly comes from phenols
- Colour develops due to the reaction of carbonyls with amino acids.
- Color formation depends upon smoke concentration, temperature and surface drying (12-15% moisture is ideal).
- Flavor in smoked product is mainly due to phenols at vapour phase, guaicol, syringol, dimethoxy phenol, etc.
- Vanillic acid gives sweet mellow flavour

Smoke deposition depends on

- More the density or velocity of air, better smoke deposition, but they are counter active to each other.
- Higher relative humidity favours deposition but reduces colour development
- Moist surface favours uptake but dry surface retards

Methods of smoking

1. *Natural air circulation:* air is regulated by opening or closing dampers
2. *Air conditioned (forced ventilation):* controlled by fan, exhaustion or recirculation of smoke. More uniform smoke, temperature and RH. More useful for cooking.

3. *Continuous smoke house:* It is developed for continuous operation with programmable processing and monitoring system.

Advantages

a) Less space occupying.

b) Labour saving.

c) Speedy processing.

d) Specific control of time, temperature and RH.

Limitations

a) Large capital investment.

b) High output (1.5-5 tonnes per hour).

Cooking during smoking

- Cooking is mostly done with smoking of meat.
- Careful control of smoking and heating is required.
- Generally cooked in heat, gas heat or electrical heat.
- Humidity kept higher for better heat transfer.
- Internal temperature should reach 70^{0}C.

Liquid smoke

- Prepared by pyrolysis of hardwood sawdust.
- Smoke is captured in water through absorption in tower.
- Recycled till desired concentration is reached.
- Solution is aged for polymerization and tar precipitation.
- Filtered through cellulose pulp to remove dissolved hydrocarbons.

Applications

1. Adding directly to meat emulsion.
2. Dipping the product in smoke solution.
3. Spraying the solution over the product.

4. Atomize into dense fog and inject into smoke house.
5. Vapourizing the liquid by putting on a hot surface.

Advantages

1. No need of a smoke generator (financial burden).
2. Process is repeatable as composition remains constant.
3. Smoke is free from particle phase (carcinogens are removed).
4. Liquid smoke creates little atmospheric pollution.
5. More throughput as application is faster.

Chemical Preservation

Preservatives

- Any substance which is capable of inhibiting, retarding or arresting the process of fermentation, acidification or other deterioration of foods.
- Permitted e.g. SO_2, $NaNO_3$, NaN^3O_2, benzoic acid (widely used), propionic acid, sorbic acid, benzoates etc.
- They should be pure, safe, no health hazards.
- Class I preservatives-Salt, sugar, acetic acid etc.
- Class II preservatives -Benzoic acid, sorbic acid, propionic acid.

Chemical preservatives, their maximum permissible limits (MPL) and functions

Name	Action	Dose
Acetic acid/lactic acid	Decontamination of carcass	1.0-2.0 % solutions
Organic acids and their salts	Reduce pH, prevent growth of bacteria, moulds, yeast, give sour taste to products	0.5 to 5 g/kg
Sulphur dioxide	Preservative in sausages	400 ppm sausage
Na/K benzoates/sorbate	Prevent growth of moulds and yeasts, suitable for pickles	0.5 to 1g/kg

Na/K meta-bisulphite (SMS, KMS)	Anti-mould, anti-yeast, prevents slime formation, suitable for sausages	0.5 to 1 g/kg
Nisin, Natamycin	Antibiotics used in cheese & canned fruits	Up to 500 ppm
BHA/BHT/Ascorbate	Antioxidants	100-200ppm

Antibiotics

- In the required concentration they do not affect flavour and color product.
- They enable to lower the processing temperature.
- Use of antibiotics is restricted because organisms may develop resistance.
- Nicin and natamycin are widely used in food preservation.
- Tetracycline - 10 to 20 ppm of tetracycline is permitted.
- Nicin - polypeptide antibiotic produced by *Streptococcus lactis* effective against G+ve and spore formers.
- Natamycin - is a polyene, effective against yeast and mold, produced by *Streptomyces natalensis.*
- Tylosin - is a macrolide acts against G+ve bacteria.

Antioxidants

- Any substance which delays or prevents the development of rancidity due to oxidation.
- Antioxidants often improve flavour in cooked meat, some prevent colour changes.
- Butylated-hydroxy anisole (BHA), Butylated-hydroxy toluene (BHT), Propylgallate (PG) are effective antioxidant.
- Permissible limits for gallate – 100 ppm, BHA & BHT – 200 ppm.

Preservatives and antioxidants may result in

- Alteration in food characteristics.
- Health problems to consumers.

- May increase sodium level and cause hyper tension.
- Nitrite - may cause accidental poisoning.
- Antibiotics - may induce microbial resistance.
- Humectants - when used in excess alter the taste and characteristics of product.

9

Processing Comminuted Meat Products

Meat Processing

- Processing refers to any treatment which brings significant changes in the physico-chemical state of meat.
- Processing invariably improves shelf life of meat.
- Many processing technique evolved in pursuit of preservation.

Purpose

- Original basis of meat processing is preservation along with developing flavourful and nutritious product.
- With refrigeration easily available, processing is mainly for convenience and variety

Importance

- In India up to 3% of total meat is processed which is up to 30% in USA.
- Excellent source of all nutrients including vitamins, minerals.

Classification

- Comminuted - sausages, nuggets, patties, balls.
- Non-comminuted - cured, smoked, canned
- Restructured - steaks, roasts, chops, cutlets etc.
- Miscellenous - barbeque, tandoori, kabab etc.

Basic Processing Steps

1. Comminution

- It refers to subdivision of raw meat to smaller pieces or particles.
- It is basically done with a mincer and fine particles are done with bowl chopper.
- This helps in uniform distribution of other ingredients and reduces toughness meat.
- The bowl rotates horizontally & slowly, knives rotate vertically at high speed.

2. Emulsification

- Meat is chopped with salt in bowl chopper for protein extraction.
- It helps in blending and distribution of all ingredients.
- Fat particle as dispersed phase and protein matrix (water with salt & protein) as continuous phase.
- Basically it is oil in water emulsion and meat proteins act as stabilizer.
- The fat droplets are above 50microns size and remain coated with protein matrix.
- Temperature should be kept low by using ice flakes.
- Sudden exposure to high temperature may cause emulsion break.

3. Forming

It is to form a specific shape of products by different technique viz. stuffing in casing for sausages, filling in molds for nuggets, loaf or patties, etc.

4. Smoking

Mainly done for special flavour both in comminuted and non-comminuted meat product.

5. Cooking

Meat and meat products are cooked by one or combination of three methods- dry heat, moist heat and microwave cooking.

Effect of cooking

1. Improve palatability by releasing and intensifying flavour compounds
2. Improves digestibility by denaturing and coagulating proteins and solubility.
3. Improves tenderness by gelatinizing collagen in connective tissue.
4. Kills microbes and increases shelf life.
5. Inactivate enzymes and reduces moisture level to extend shelf life.

Doneness: the intensity of cooking

- Rare done: 58 to 60°C pink colour
- Medium rare: 66 to 68°C pinkish.
- Medium done: 73 to75°C Brownish/greyish
- Well done: 80 to 82°C Brown/grey

Methods of Cooking

I. **Dry heating:** suitable for tender cuts-pork chops, leg and chops of lamb, ground meats etc. Yield is high due to less shrinkage. This include broiling, roasting, frying.

   a) *Broiling:* is done in electric or gas oven or in charcoal.

   b) *Roasting:* in hot air oven or roasting pan, good for tender cuts; pork shoulder and loin, shoulder, rack or loin of lamb. It gives good browning and flavour.The roast piece, at least 8cm thick.

   c) *Frying:* may be deep or shallow pan frying, suitable for thin cuts like mutton chops, sliced steaks, chicken pieces.

II. **Moist heating**: Recommended for relatively tough cuts. Hot water or steam remains in contact so moisture loss is less. Pressure cooking, steaming, simmering are moist cooking.

   a) *Pressure cooking:* temperature is high facilitates tenderization of tough meats.

   b) *Steaming:* Efficient heating but less then pressure cooking.

c) *Simmering:* is cooking at 70°c in hot water for long time.

d) *Stewing:* is first brown in fat/oil then cook in water at simmering by covering, product will be tender and juicy.

Braising: Combination of dry heat and moist heat. First fried in oil then water is added and cooked with lid.

III. **Microwave cooking**:

- High frequency, non ionising electromagnetic waves, generated by vacuum tube (magnetron).
- Microwave frequencies viz. 915 and 2450 megahertz are commonly used.
- The microwave penetrates the food from all directions causing vibrations in food particles leading to frictions, heating and cooking.
- It takes only 25% of time of normal cooking.
- Glass, pottery, wood and paper vessels are used, metal container not suitable.
- No nutritional damage to protein, lipid and vitamins.

Additional techniques in meat processing

Meat extension: Several non-meat ingredients are used in meat products, generally they are termed as extenders; specifically they are referred as fillers, emulsifiers, binders, depending on their purpose and properties.

Purpose

- Improve water binding, emulsion stability, flavour and sliceability
- Reduce shrinkage and cost.
- *Binders:* Binds water and fat- dried milk, wheat flour, soy flour.
- *Fillers:* binds only water, mashed potato, corn, rice etc.
- *Emulsifier/stabilizer:* Improve the emulsification /stabilization eg. carageenan, egg yolk, whole egg etc.

Pre-blending: Mixing of the curing ingredients with minced meat well in advance. This allows better extraction of proteins and makes more stable emulsion, especially in case of tough meat.

Hot processing: Pre-rigor processing of carcass without chilling. Pre-rigor meat has better functional properties, more actin and myosin extracted. There is improvement in the cooking yield and sensory quality of the product.

Ingredients for meat processing

Meat

- The primary ingredient, varies in functional properties and composition.
- Mainly skeletal muscle, low value cuts and organ meats are used to reduce cost.
- Binding ability is important to hold meat pieces, stabilize fat and water.

Non-meat ingredients

1. **Water:** Helps in mixing, dissolving and distribution of other ingredients; Controls temperature, improves juiciness and yield.
2. **Curing ingredients:** Salt, sugar, phosphate, nitrite; plays major role in protein extraction, emulsification, colour, flavour and as antioxidants. (See details in Chapter 8, Curing section).
3. **Binders, fillers, extenders:** Used to improve emulsion stability, WHC, yield, juiciness and flavour and to reduce cost.
4. **Seasonings:** Any ingredient added to improve or modify the flavour of meat products.eg, onion-ginger-garlic paste, dry spices mix, MSG.

Comminuted Meat Product

Sausages

- Sausage term was derived from the latin word 'salsus' meaning salt.
- It was literally coined to refer to ground meat which was salted and stuffed in animal casings.
- Presently, sausages may be defined as a meat product which is prepared from minced and seasoned meat and formed into cylindrical shape by natural or synthetic casings.

- Though sausages originated in the western world, these products acquired universal popularity due to variety and convenience to the consumers.
- Sausages are economical also because these are generally prepared from cheaper cuts of meat and by-product of industry.

Classification

Sausages are available in large number of varying kinds and difficult to classify. The popular classification is :

i) *Based on degree of chopping:* coarse ground sausage, Emulsion type sausage.

ii) *Based on moisture content:* dry sausage, semidry sausage.

iii) *Based on cooking:* fresh sausage, smoked uncooked sausage, cooked sausage.

iv) *Based on fermentation:* fermented sausage, non-fermented sausage.

Processing steps

i) *Grinding or mincing* Lean meat and fat are minced separately in a meat mincer. The choice of mincer plate or sieve depends on the type of meat.

ii) *Mixing* Meat and fat to be used for the preparation of coarse ground sausage are mixed uniformly in a mixer. Extender, condiments and spices should also be run in the mixer for even distribution.

iii) *Chopping and emulsifying*: (As discussed earlier).

iv) *Stuffing* Sausage emulsion or better is taken to stuffer for extrusion into casings. The casings are first collected on the stuffing horn or nozzle and released to coincide with the extrusion.

v) *Linking and tying* In small sausages, the encased mass is twisted to produce links either manually or mechanically whereas in large sausages, the encased mass is tied with thread at regular intervals.

vi) *Smoking and cooking* Sausages links are hung on the smokehouse trolley and transferred to smokehouse. The temperature of smokehouse is usually maintained at 68-70°C which is enough for coagulation of sausages emulsion, cooking and requisite drying of sausages.

vii) *Chilling* The cooked product is showered with chilled water to an internal temperature of about 4°C.

viii) *Peeling and packaging* While artificial or synthetic casings are peeled off before the product is packed, small sized natural casings need not to be removed. The product is generally unit packed for retail outlets.

Formulation of some sausages with special features

i) Fresh pork sausages (coarse ground type)

Ingredients	*Quantity*
Lean pork trimmings	35.0 kg
Back fat	15.0 kg
Table salt	1.0 kg
White pepper	125.0 kg
Sugar	75.0 kg
Ginger powder	15.0 kg

ii) Frankfurters (Cured, emulsion type)

Ingredients	*Quantity*
Beef trimmings	30.0 kg
Pork trimmings (50/50)	20.0 kg
Ice flakes	15.0 kg
Table salt	1.2 kg
White pepper	110.0 g
Nutmeg	25.0 g
Cardamom	25.0 g
Ginger powder	25.0 g
Monosodium glutamate (MSG)	25.0 g
Sodium erythorbate	20.0 g
Sodium nitrite	7.5 g

iii) Salami (fresh, emulsion type)

Ingredients	*Quantity*
Pork trimmings (50-50)	20.0kg
Pork cheek meat	10.0 kg
Pork hearts	10.0 kg
Pork stomachs	5.0 kg
Ice flakes	5.0 kg
Table salt	1.2 kg
Black pepper	115.0g
Sodium erythorbate	25.0 g
Garlic powder	25.0 g
Sodium nitrite	5.0 g

Batter is stuffed in broader casings, usually dried cattle oesophagus and hanged for 2 days at 4°C. It is smoked and cooked simultaneously in India.

vii) *Bologna:* It is an emulsion type sausage prepared from the meat of old animals.

viii) *Hot dog:* It is a fairly spicy sausage in broader casings, usually in weasand.

ix) *Mortadella:* It is dry sausage prepared in cattle bladder or artificial broader casings.

Other Comminuted Meat Products

1. Meat patties

- A popular comminuted meat products generally used in burger, roll or sandwich.
- Some people prefer to consume it with tomato sauce or chutney as snack.
- It is ground or emulsion based product containing up to 30% fat.
- Lean meat is minced twice through 4 mm plate of mincer.
- Mix with other ingredients in food mixer or make emulsion in bowl chopper.

- Prepare patties of 70-80 mm diameter and 15-20 mm thickness with a mould.
- Raw patties may be frozen or cooked in preheated oven at 160ºC for 40 minutes.
- The patties are cooled and consumer packed.

A standard formulation of patties

Ingredients	*Percentage*
Lean meat	65
Fat	15
Table salt	2
Texturised soy protein	10
Condiments	6.5
Dry spices	1.5

2. Meat nuggets

- It is ready to eat emulsion type meat product with a similar recipe of sausage/balls.
- Meat emulsion is prepared in the same way as discussed earlier.
- The emulsion is filled in rectangular mould and cooked in steam/ hot water.
- The rectangular block obtained after cooking is cut into pieces.
- The product is packed pouches and can be stored at 4ºC for a week.
- It can be used as snack or side dish after shallow frying before serving.

A standard recipe for Nuggets

Ingredients	**Percentage**
Lean pork	65
Pork back fat	15
Ice flakes	5
Table salt	2
Refined wheat flour	7.5
Skim milk powder	4
Dry spices	1.5
Sodium nitrite	150 ppm

3. Meat balls

- The batter is prepared by mixing ground meat with fat, bread crumb, salt, condiments and spices in a food mixer.
- The batter of 15-20 g are rolled into balls manually or mechanically.
- These are either stored raw or deep fat fried in oil at 135°C for 3-4 minutes.
- Can be cooked in hot water at 80°C for 20 minutes.
- These are packed in polyethylene pouches and kept in 4°C for a week.
- The balls can be used as snack or to prepare in gravy for rice or bread.

4. Meat loaves

- Ready-to-eat comminuted meat product prepared from ground meat or emulsion.
- Formulation and batter making is almost similar to nuggets or sausages
- The meat batter is filled in aluminium or steel mould of desired shape.
- Cook in hot air oven at 165°C for 2.5-3 hours at internal temperature of 70°C.
- Remove loaves and pack as such or after slicing into desired thickness.
- Slices are best used in making sandwitches.

5. Fermented meat products

- Fermented meat products rely on microbial fermentation and dehydration to develop their specified flavour and texture.
- In the production of fermented meat products, we add selected bacterial culture to the minced meat.
- These are called starter culture, available commercially.
- These contain microorganisms like *Lactobacillus, Pediococcus, Lactococcus* and *Micrococcus.*

- After addition of starter culture to minced meat, mixture is kept at specific temperature and humidity for a specified period.
- This allows maximum growth of added bacteria, the process is called fermentation. During fermentation bacteria utilize sugar and produce lactic acid, which causes decrease in pH.
- After completion of fermentation, product is dried to specific moisture level. After drying, products are cooked or smoked.

Characteristics of fermented meat products

- Fermentation of meat involves lowering of pH due to conversion of added sugar to lactic acid by large number of lactic acid bacteria.
- Fermented meat products have characteristic flavour, taste and texture.
- The fermented meat products have very long shelf life.
- Fermented products can be of ground type, emulsified or cured and smoked products.

Longer shelf life of fermented meat products is due to

- Lower pH
- Lower moisture content and thus lower water activity
- Competitive bacteria (large number of LAB prevents growth of spoilage bacteria).

Preparation of fermented meat products

Inoculation: Minced meat and different ingredients are mixed and then lactic acid bacteria (starter culture) are added.

Fermentation: After inoculation, mixer is stuffed into casings and allowed to ferment for 1 to 4 days at 18 to 43°C and 70 to 80% relative humidity.

Drying: After fermentation is complete, products are dried to the desired moisture level.

Semi-dry sausages having moisture content between 40 to 50 per cent require ageing or drying up to 5 days.

Dry sausages having moisture content between 30 to 40 per cent are placed in drying chamber up to 10 days

Storage: Dry sausages do not require refrigerated storage. However, semidry sausages require refrigeration to prevent microbial spoilage.

□□□

10

Processing Non-comminuted Meat Products

Cured and Smoked Meat Products

- All meat products belonging to this class are cured, some of them are smoked.
- The primal cuts of pork especially ham and bacon usually cured and smoked.
- Nowadays cooking also done during smoking except for country ham.

Processing of hams

- Most hams are processed in three steps- curing, smoking and cooking.
- Most commercial hams are pickle cured, by artery pumping or stitch pumping to 10% of the weight.
- Best colour and flavour obtained by keeping the hams in cover pickle at 4°C for 5 days.
- Then hams are shifted to smoke chamber at 75-85°C temperature and 30-40% relative humidity for 5-6 hours.

A typical curing solution (65°salometer)

Ingredient	Percent	Quantity
Salt	25	250g
Sugar	10	100g
NaNo3	0.2	2g
TSPP	0.5	5G
Water		1000ml

Advantages of cover pickle

- Better colour development and colour stability
- More uniform distribution of salt
- Better flavour and water binding
- Fewer uncured spots

Country hams

- It is dry cured by rubbing at the rate of 30g per kg of ham on 1st, 5th and 10^{th}day.
- Curing is allowed to take place under refrigeration at a relative humidity of 70-90% for 30-40 days during which hams are overhauled at least three times,
- Aging is done for 6-9 months at a temperature of 20-30°C and relative humidity of 50-60%.
- Smoking is done at low temperature for 2-3 days till the hams become amber coloured.
- Salty, somewhat dry, rather hard, highly flavoured.
- Shrinkage up to 18% during processing.
- Final moisture 50-60%, salt 4.5-5.5%.
- Lean ham dark red & very firm, fat quite yellow.
- Flavor intense and distinctive.

Cooked ham

- These hams are deboned and cured in pickle but smoking is not done.
- Cured hams are stuffed into metal moulds and cooked in water at 75-85°C for 2-3 hours.
- After cooking, the moulds are chilled in water tank maintained at 0°C for 12 hours.
- These hams are then sliced and packed.

Commercial ham preparation

Ham (Cut and trimmed)

↓

Inject cure solution (10% of gross wt)

↓

Hold for 24hrs at 4°C

↓

Hold in cover pickle (at 2-4°C for 3-7 days

↓

Smoking and cooking

↓

(Start at 60°C, 70°C for 2hrs, up to 82°C)

↓

Slicing

↓

Packaging

Processing of bacon

- Pork bellies are generally processed as cured and smoked bacon.
- Green bellies are first cleared of rind and stitch pumped with a curing pickle.
- Transfer to smoke chamber at 60-65°C, RH 30-40% for smoking and cooking.
- The cooking time depends on the size, internal temperature must be 55°C.
- Then bacon is chilled to 0°C and pressed to get proper shape and facilitate slicing,
- Bacon blocks are now sliced to 5-7 mm thickness.
- The slices may be packed MAP if long term storage is desired.

Preparation of bacon

Pig bellies
↓
Curing (pickle injection at 10%
↓
Combing (pierce with multiple hanger)
↓
Brine curing 3-4 days
↓
Smoking and cooking
↓
Chilling
↓
Pressing
↓
Slicing
↓
Packaging

Canned Meat Products

Luncheon meat

- It is a canned product usually prepared from pork along with some cereals.
- Contains pork up to 80% and pork fat up to 30% in the finished product.
- Added water up to 3% and cereals up to 7% of the total formulation.
- Meat and fat are ground in meat mincer and batter is prepared in bowl chopper.
- Batter is maintained at 4°C and then filled compactly in cans.
- Cans are sealed under vacuum and sterilized in retorts at 121°C for 75 minutes.
- Cans are cooled with cold water shower until it reaches 38°C.
- Luncheon meat is stable at ambient temperature for a period of two years.

Typical formulation

Lean pork	-	67 %
Pork back fat	-	15 %
Ice Flakes	-	3 %
Salt	-	2.5%
Dextrose	-	1.5 %
Refined wheat flour	-	5 %
Condiments	-	4.75
Dry spices	-	1.5 %
Sodium nitrate	-	150 ppm.

Canned poultry

- Well fleshed, mature chicken with similar age and conformation.
- Precooking at 60°C for 15 min
- Filling of precooked bird into the can keeping space at the top.
- Thermal Exhaustion by passing through steam, sometimes vacuum closing
- Seaming -usually done by double seaming machine
- Washing with detergent spray to remove grease
- Retort processing at 116°C for 75 min or 121°C for 65 min)
- Cooling by slowly reducing pressure.
- Storage at 20°C, RH 30-40% should be maintained.

Miscellaneous Meat Products

Restructured meat products

- Restructuring is a processing technique used for developing convenience products.
- It facilitates to develop more palatable products from buffalo meat, pork, and from chicken.
- Restructured meat generally prepared by first deforming meat and again reforming into different form
- Chunking/flaking/tearing and mixing by tumbling or messaging.

Procedure

Deboned minced meat
↓
Mixing with all ingredients
↓
Tumbling using home mixer grinder
↓
Filling in a stainless steel mould
↓
Keeping overnight in refrigerator (4±1°C)
↓
Cooking in water at 90°C for 45 minutes
↓
Cooling and chilling (4±1°C) for overnight
↓
Opening and slicing
↓
Packing and storage

Enrobed meat products

- Enrobing is a method by which food material is coated with edible coating materials in the form of batter.
- Enrobing adds the value of a product by improving eating quality such as texture, juiciness and nutritive value.
- Highly acceptable enrobed pork patties have been made using Bengal gram flour, refined wheat flour and corn flour as coating materials.
- Enrobed pork patties can be kept more than 28 days at refrigeration (4±1°C) under aerobic packaging condition.

Traditional Meat Products

- Traditional meat products getting popularity in many western countries.
- Indigenous meat products are unique in flavor and ease of preparation.
- They are becoming value added convenience products of good palatability.
- Popular indigenous meat products are meat pickle, kebab, tikka and kofta.

Meat pickle

Formulation of meat pickle

Ingredient	*Percent*	*Quantity*
Meat chunks (boneless)	100	1000g
Salt	4	40g
Dry spice mix	4	40g
Green condiments	10	100g
Mustard oil	20	200ml
Acetic acid	1	10ml

Preparation of meat pickle

Deboned Meat
↓
Clean and make into small pieces
↓
Presalting (with 50% salt)
↓
Keep it for 1 to 2 hours
↓
Pressure cook the meat for 20 minutes
↓
Separate the cooked meat from the broth
↓
Frying Pieces in oil till golden brown
↓
Straining and separation of fried pieces
↓
Fry the condiments and spices in the same oil
↓
Add the fried meat pieces
↓
Continue cooking for 2-3 minutes
↓
Cooling
↓
Add acetic acid (1%)
↓
Mix well
↓
Packing and storing

Meat kabab

- There are different varieties of *kababs* which are popular in India.
- *Kababs* are made either from ground meat or from chunks.
- Generally kababs have been made from red meats.
- Three popular kababs are *Seekh kabab*, *Shami kabab* and *Boti kabab*.
- Common ingredients salt, lime juice, Bengal gram paste, egg, dry spice mix, green chilies, garlic, ginger and cream.
- Proportion of ingredients varies with the kind of kabab.
- Binders such as wheat flour and egg liquid added at 3% and 5% levels respectively.
- The main steps involved in the preparation of kababs are marination and cooking.

Formulation

Minced meat	100
Egg liquid	5
Minced fat/Oil	5
Onion chopped	5
Green chilly	2
Ginger	2
Garlic	1
Spice mix	3
Wheat flour	3
Salt	1.5

Preparation

1. Mix the lightly beaten egg and fat with the minced meat in a bowl.
2. Mix spices, salt and chopped onion, chilly, ginger, garlic and wheat flour to get a dough
3. Oil your fingers and the skewers.
4. Wrap the dough around the skewers in cigar shapes.

5. Brush the meat with oil and cook under a moderate grill until evenly browned.
6. Serve garnished with lemon, onion and tomato slices.
7. Seekh-kabab gives a blend of meat and smoke flavour.

Tandoori chicken

- Dry cooked with minimum spices, without oil in conventional type tandoor oven.
- Broilers of 5-6 weeks old are suitable for tandoori chicken.

Formulation of marinate (spice mix)

Ingredients	Parts
Curd	100
Garlic paste	7
Ginger paste	7
Lemon juice	5
Salt	5
Chilli powder	3
Turmeric powder	0.4

Procedure

- Skinless dressed chicken - leg and breast muscles incised.
- Marinate for 1-2 hours with spice mix.
- Drain excess spice mix and insert long iron rods into marinated chicken for cooking.
- Initially cook for 10 minutes then apply butter and cook for 10 more minutes.
- Now the product is ready for serving.

Chicken soup powder

- Soup powders prepared from vegetables, meat, fish, chicken etc.
- These are rich in dietary constituents like protein, vitamin, fat and minerals.

- Fishes of low economic value can very well be used for preparing soup powder.
- The soup powders are generally prepared by freeze drying.

Chicken soup preparation

Boneless chicken
↓
Cut into pieces
↓
Oil taken in pressure pan
↓
Pour the pieces and condiments
↓
Fried for sometime
↓
Add spices, salt
↓
Add water
↓
Pressure-cooked for 30 minutes (15 psi)
↓
Filtered through clean, fine muslin cloth
↓
Chicken soup

❑❑❑

11

Packaging of Meat and Meat Products

Packaging refers to the scientific method of containing a food for optimum protection till it reaches the ultimate consumer. In modern terms, packaging is considered as a marketing tool. Proper packaging helps in maintaining the quality of the product during storage, transport and provides the convenience for easy handling.

The function of packaging for fresh meat

1. To prevent moisture loss during storage
2. To offer meat in the most desirable colour
3. To prevent microbial contamination
4. To prevent foreign odour absorption
5. To prevent lipid oxidation

Characteristics of packaging films

Flexibility, mechanical strength, light weight, odourless, hygienic, harmless, easy recycling, resistance to hot and cold temperatures, resistance to oil and fats, good barrier properties against gases, sealing capability & low-cost.

Packaging materials and forms

Rigid: Glass containers, metal cans, composite containers, aerosol containers, rigid plastic packages

Semi-rigid: Aluminium containers, Set-up paper board boxes, folding paper board cartons

Flexible films: Cellophane, cellulose acetate, polyethylene (HDPE & LDPE), polypropylene, polyamide, polyester, polyvinyl chloride, polyvinylidene chloride, polyvinyl acetate and polyvinyl alcohols.

New films: Amylase films (edible), ionomers like surlyn A, ethylene vinyl acetate copolymers, polypropylene copolymers, co-extruded films, aluminium foils.

Flexible package forms: Wrappers, preformed bags or envelopes, pouches, collapsible tubes.

Packaging Techniques for Fresh Meat

- Fresh meat is highly perishable, prone to dehydration & oxidation.
- Thus the packaging should be able to minimise these two.
- Fresh meat has characteristic colour, texture and flavour which are to be protected.
- Materials should withstand freezing and be impermeable to odour & flavour.
- Major materials used are: LDPE (200-300gauge), Polyester/PE, Polyamide/PE laminated film, cryovac (PVC, PVDC copolymer).

A. Overwraps

- Done with thermoplastic films having excellent optical properties.
- LDPE is the cheapest and widely used.
- Rubber HCl, Nylon, plasticised PVC can also be used.
- Cellophane coated with nitrocellulose or P.E cases can be used for irregular shape.
- The uncoated side should contact the meat.

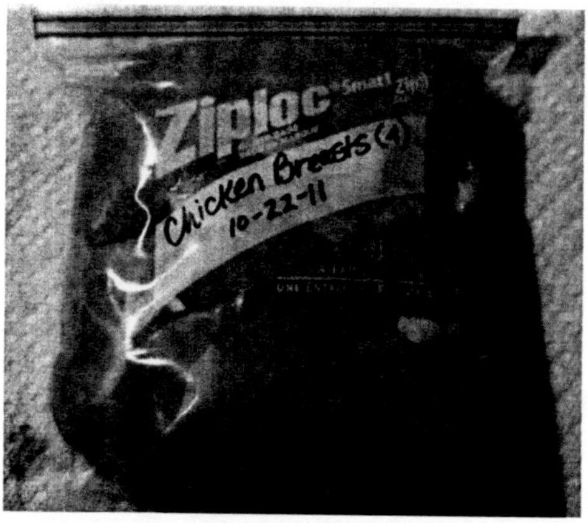

Fresh Chicken

B. Tray with-overwrap

- The common packages for fresh meat cuts in the Western countries
- Polystyrene foam or clear plastic trays over-wrapped with a thin thermoplastic film.
- Tray gives an appealing background.
- Meat has a shelf life of 10 days but bright red colour remains only for 5 days.

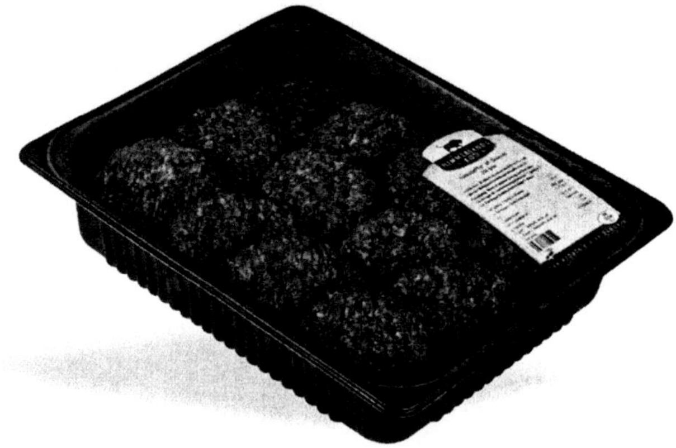

Tray with-overwrap

C. Shrink film overwrap

- These films shrink on exposure to hot air or hot water for a few seconds.
- They have good moisture barrier and strength.
- Used for wrapping large and uneven cuts of fresh meat.
- Shrink film offers neat appearance, contour of package & easy handling.
- They can be used for freezing quarters.
- Heat shrinkable PP, irradiated PE, PVDC can be used for this purpose.

D. Vacuum packaging (VAP)

- This is for long term storage of primal and sub-primal cuts of buffalo and beef.
- Ensures shelf-life of 8 - 10 weeks at 0^0C.
- Vacuum shrink packaging is suitable for storage and transport of carcasses & quarters for export.
- Vacuum packaging is done in laminates or co-extruded films.
- Typical laminates are: Aluminium foil/PE, Polyester/PE, Polyamide/PE, PVDC/Polyester/PE.

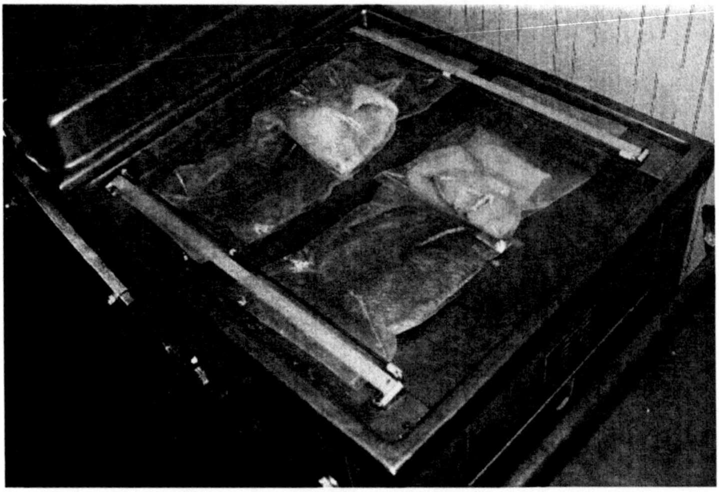

Vaccum packaging

E. Modified atmosphere packaging (MAP)

- Atmosphere inside the package (air composition) is modified to extend the shelf-life of meat while retaining its colour, flavour and weight.
- Air is replaced with suitable concentration of nitrogen, oxygen & CO_2.
- Different meats have different requirements.
- Buffalo and beef meat need high oxygen content, pork needs less oxygen due to more fat.
- Nitrogen serves as inert filler.

Packaging of Meat Products

A. Frozen meat products

- Both raw and pre-cooked meat can be frozen e.g. Patties, Hamburger, Nuggets etc.
- Precooked frozen meat products are generally prone to oxidation and desiccation.
- For packaging tandoori, barbeque and meat in gravy HDPE or aluminium is used.
- For hamburger, hot dog a double protection is needed (e.g. Glassine)
- Glassine is wrapped over the product and is pressed & frozen
- When needed, the glassine bag is heated to recover the hamburger or hot dog.

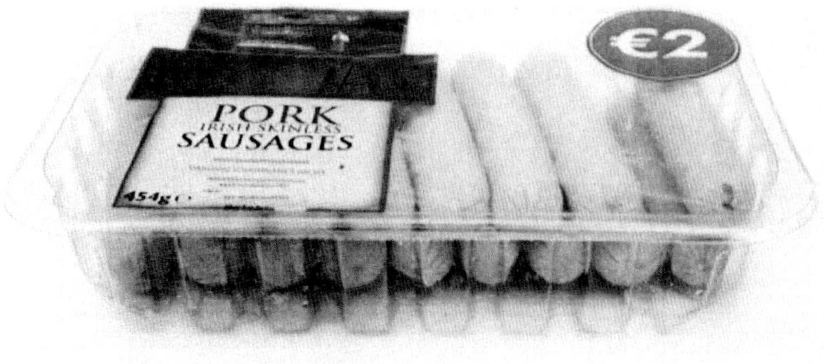

Sausages

B. Cured meat

- Packaging should prevent dehydration, fading of pink colour, flavour loss and microbial contamination
- For Short term packaging, plastic film overwraps and shrink films are used
- Chub packs are used - ground cured meat is filled in tubes of PE/Cellophane and the ends are twisted.
- For long term storage - vacuum packaging or MAP is done.
- Shelf life is 2-3 months at 4^0C and 6 months at -18^0C in vacuum packing.

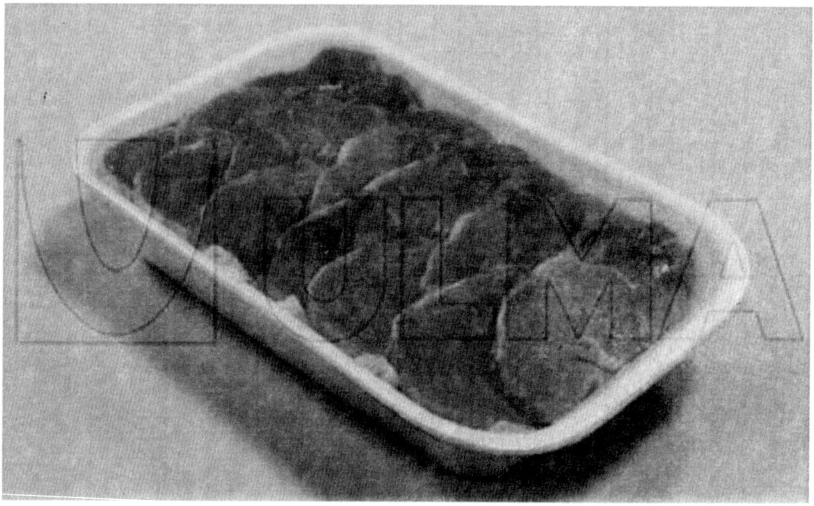

Cured meat

C. Dehydrated meat products

- These are meat products prepared for military ration and space travel.
- It can be done by hot air drying or freeze drying followed by packaging.
- For compressed bar of dehydrated minced meat - Paper/Al foil, vacuum sealing in metal cans, packaging in metal cans with nitrogen can be done.
- For vacuum pack and MAP - Polyester/Al foil/PE , Polyamide/ Al foil/PE can be used.

D. Thermo processed meat products

- Products like meat balls, corned beef, boneless chicken, meat soup etc. are sealed in cans.
- Most cooked meats are canned & have a storage life of 1-2 years.
- Aluminium cans, tin cans can be used.
- Cans are lined internally with epoxides.
- Packing can be done in retort pouches of Polyester/Al foil/PP.

Modern Packaging System

1. Antimicrobial packaging

- To improve safety and to delay spoilage by use of antibacterial sprays or dips.
- Bactericidal agents into meat may inactivate the active compounds.
- Extends shelf life and maintain product quality and safety.
- Examples are acid anhydride, alcohols, bacteriocins, chelators, enzymes, organic acids and polysaccharides.

2. Active packaging

- Incorporation of additives in packaging for extending meat product quality and shelf-life.
- Allows packages to interact with food and play a dynamic role in the food preservation.
- Delays oxidation and controls respiration, microbial growth and moisture migration.
- CO2 absorbers and emitters, odour absorbers, ethylene removers and aroma emitters.
- Purge control is most successful e.g. drip absorbing pad in poultry industry.

3. Intelligent packaging

- Monitors the condition of packaged foods to give information about the quality of the packaged food during transport and storage.
- Used as indicators of freshness, time-temperature (TTI).
- Radio frequency identification (RFID) is used in meat and meat products.
- This smart device may be incorporated in packages.

❏❏❏

12

Eating Quality and Sensory Evaluation

Eating Quality of Meat Food Products

The important eating quality attributes are

1. Appearance & Colour
2. Texture & Tenderness
3. Flavour
4. Juiciness

Knowledge of these attributes is important for their subjective & objective assessment.

1. Appearance and colour

- Appearance is a wider term than colour.
- Appearance & colour have a definite appeal for the consumer or panellist.
- The colour of fresh meat is species specific, it depends on meat pigment (myoglobin).
- The final colour of cooked meat is dependent upon the pigment changes brought about by temperature, time & method of cooking.
- The brown colour of thoroughly cooked meat is due to denaturation of heme pigments & polymerisation of some proteins & fats.

2. Texture and tenderness

- Most important attribute for acceptance of meat.
- Perceived by senses of touch, sight & hearing.

- Different components of texture includes:
  - i) *Mechanical component*: which relates to the effect of stress, e.g. hard, brittle, gummy, chewy, elastic, cohesive etc.
  - ii) *Geographical component*: which relates to size, shape & arrangement of fibres in meat, e.g. coarse, grainy, gritty, fibrous etc.
  - iii) *Moisture & fat perception of meat*: e.g. greasy, oily, watery, dry, moist etc.

Factors considered on tenderness

1. Ease with which teeth sink into meat.
2. Ease with which meat breaks into fragments.
3. Leftover residue after chewing.

3. Flavour

- It is a complex sensation comprising mainly taste & odour.
- It is sensed jointly by the oral & olfactory senses. Flavour is more after cooking & is very important for acceptability.
- When cooked meat is stored for a long time, fat oxidation takes place yielding *warmed-over-flavour*.

4. Juiciness

- Juiciness of cooked meat comprises of two components:

First impression of juiciness comes from rapid release of meat fluids during initial chews.

Sustained juiciness: due to slow release of serum & stimulatory effect of fat on salivation.

- A good quality meat is more juicy than that of poor quality because of higher content of intramuscular fat.
- Cooking temperature has a profound effect on juiciness.
- Shrinkage on cooking is inversely related to juiciness.
- Juiciness & tenderness are closely related. In tender meat, the juices are quickly released & left over residue is less.

5. Overall acceptability

Indicates general aspect in total, but tenderness & flavour plays more important role.

Sensory evaluation

Sensory evaluation is the scientific way of evaluation of meat products through use of human senses such as smell, taste, touch, temperature etc. Human senses act as biological detector, which can perceive taste, smell etc.

Applications of sensory analysis in meat science

1. Quality control of meat and meat products,
2. New product development
3. Analysis of competitive products
4. Product shelf life studies
5. Market level consumer tests
6. Aroma research etc.

Advantage: Only the human sensory perception can properly assess all attributes & the total impression of a food product.

Consumer panel

It is for knowing likes or dislikes, preferences and acceptability using untrained panels.

- Consists of 100 or more persons drawn from the local population.
- They need not have any formal education or training.
- It can be conducted at any central location-supermarket, consumers' homes.
- Panellists can easily be involved in ranking test or hedonic score test.

In-house panels are commonly used before true consumer panel. The in-house panels consists of 30-50 untrained people from the organization, who use the product and similar to the target consumer. These results are not good for predicting product performance.

Specialized Panel

- Product oriented evaluation is done by specialised panel.
- Sensory panel members are selected on the basis of general health, appetite, sensitivity, willingness, availability, etc.
- Their sensitivity is tested by conducting recognition test & threshold test for four basic tastes (sweet, salty, sour & bitter).
- Then they are trained about meat traits.
- These small numbers of trained panellists use their senses as biological detectors & can identify even minor differences in the eating quality.
- The data obtained from specialised as well as consumer panel is statistically analysed to enable proper interpretation & application of results.

Training of sensory panelists

- The goal is to familiarize with test procedures.
- To improve ability to recognize/identify sensory attributes.
- To improve sensitivity and memory for sensory attributes ultimately to have precise and consistent judgments.

Number of panellists- depends on (a) familiarity with the product and procedures, (b) Expected differences between products (c) 20% extra, for drop out due to many reasons.

First Session: Educate about general biology of muscle foods viz. muscle fibre structure, connective tissue, fat coating etc.

- How the Olfactory senses work?
- Four basic tastes, their location in tongue.
- Sensory attributes of meat & meat products.

Main Sessions: To familiarize panellists with test procedures. Techniques to be presented are :

- How to chew a sample?
- How to expectorate the sample–vs–swallowing.

- How to rinse mouth between each sample.
- Methods of evaluation – viz. -scale to be used, - anchor points for the scale, - score sheet, terminology to be used.

The type of training needed for panellist depends on the objectives of the study. Muscle foods are evaluated mainly by two types of sensory panels. That is difference testing or descriptive testing. Selection of panellists and amount of training required varies with the type of sensory task.

- Generally they are required to pass through the threshold test for 4 basic tastes.
- Through training and experience they understand judging techniques and critical analysis.
- For meat products panellist should develop the ability to judge one attribute at a time without the influence of other attributes.

General guidelines for training

1. Present reference sample for each attribute.
2. Concentrate on one attribute in a session till they are familiar with it.
3. Anchor points on the scale for each attribute and how to scale within attribute.
4. Panellists should score individually, then discuss in a group.
5. Panel leader gives overall score.
6. Panellists should re-evaluate to familiarize.
7. Continue & repeat till consistent results are obtained among panellists.
8. Length of training depends on type of panel, number of attributes, previous experience.

Sensory panel room

1. Panel area should be separated from sample preparation area, free from external & cooking odours.
2. Sample transfer mechanism avoiding odour transfer.

3. Odours from other panellists to be minimized e.g. cosmetics, tobacco etc., (on that day avoid hand cream, hair/body spray, lotion etc.).
4. Sinks, drain pipe, water odour avoid, (deionised or double distilled).
5. Materials non porous, no odours, neutral colour (off white) no pattern, not collect dirt.
6. Room temperature 22-24^{0}C, RH-45-55%.
7. Minimize noise level- external (traffic) or internal.
8. No communication (visual or oral) between panellists.
9. Consistent & appropriate light – 70-80 ft/candle, shadowless for meat foods.
10. Minimize physical discomfort - seating, space etc.
11. Unbiased presentation of samples.
12. Preparation of samples affect sensory attributes e.g. cooking method, serving temperature, holding time, interval from cooking to serving, etc.

Time of Taste: Depends upon the sample

1. Taste subjects are more sensitive when they are hungry.
2. Lunch time should be avoided for taste panel.
3. For meat, fish etc., ideal time is late morning, afternoon, at least 1.5 hr after lunch.
4. Tea /Coffee may be given after breakfast or 1/2hr after lunch.

In other way sensory evaluation can be two types (i) Product oriented and (ii) Consumer oriented.

Preparation and Presentation of Samples

1. Cooking method, serving temperature, humidity etc.
2. Degree of doneness, time length and interval from cooking holding period & temperature.
3. Containers used for storing and preparing.

4. Size or quantity of sample:
   - for whole muscle product (steaks, chops, roasts) $1.27cm^3$.
   - ground meat product 1.27 or 2.54 cm^2.
   - for texture evaluation of frankfurters – a whole piece.
   - for flavour evaluation of sausages a 2.54 cm section.
5. Temperature of sample can affect sensory perception.
6. Samples should have 3 digit random code (to avoid subconscious selection).
7. Use glass or white glazed china for presentation, (to eliminate aromatics or visual attribute on sample).
8. Plastics should be opaque, free from odours and neutral in colour.
9. Samples served in random order to avoid order effect (1st sample ranked high or low).

Sensory Evaluation Methods

Objective methods

- They involve use of instruments such as Instron/Texturometer, Warner Bratzler shear Press, Flavour Analyzers, Hunter colour Lab/Colorimeter etc. for above-mentioned sensory characteristics.

Subjective methods

These methods include perception through human senses. It involves the specialized panel or consumer panel for testing the sensory attributes of meat and meat products.

Recognition and Threshold tests: This test is used for training of the panel members for making them familiar to four basic tastes. The serial dilutions in ascending order of 0.01% of all the four tastes (cane sugar-sweet; sodium chloride-salty; tartaric acid/citric acid-sourness; caffeine-bitterness) are prepared.

Ranking test: The objective is to select one or two best samples out of all tested samples. A series of test samples are provided in an ascending or descending order of intensity of specific characteristics. The trainee receives a random order of sample and is asked to rank the samples in order of increasing intensity.

Hedonic scaling: In hedonic scaling, effective responses of like and dislikes are measured on a rating scale. Most popular are 8-point or 9-point Hedonic scale, where 8 or 9 = like extremely and 1 = dislike extremely.

Difference test

Paired difference test: In this test, two samples are provided and the analysis is done for a single attribute. The trainee has to identify the sample having more intensity of the specified attribute.

Duo-trio test: In this test, three samples are presented to trainee. One of them is reference sample and other two are coded samples. The trainee has to identify that among the coded samples, which one is similar or different to reference sample.

Triangle test: In this test, three coded samples are provided to trainee and he has to identify which two samples are same or different from the other sample.

❑❑❑

13

Meat Species Identification

- Adulteration of meat involves substitution of costly or superior quality with cheaper, undesirable or inferior quality meat.
- It is a fraudulent practice that is objectionable on the grounds of health, religion and economics.
- It is punishable under prevention of food adulteration act, 1955.
- The substitutions generally practiced are mutton for goat meat (chevon), beef for buffalo meat, rabbit meat for chicken etc.
- The instances of dog or cat meat or even veal as goat meat have also come to light.

Methods for Recognition of Fraudulent Substitution or Adulteration

Methods/techniques

Various methods have been developed for identification of species origin of meat and meat products. These include-

1. Anatomical methods
2. Physical methods
3. Chemical methods
4. Electrophoretic methods
5. Biological methods
6. Molecular biology methods

1. Anatomical methods

i) Rib number

Paired ribs vary in number in different species of animal

S.No.	Species	Ribs in pairs	Sternal ribs
1	Ox	13	8
2	Pig	14-15	7
3	Sheep and Goat	13	8
4	Horse	18	8
5	Dog	13	9

ii) Characteristics of long bones

S.No.	Bone	Species	Characteristics
1	Scapula	Sheep	Short and broad, superior spine thick and bent back.
		Goat	Possesses distinct neck spine, straight and narrow.
2	Radius	Sheep	1.25 times length of metacarpus.
		Goat	Twice the length of metacarpus.
3	Ulna	Horse	Extends only ½ the length of radius.
		Ox	Extends and articulates with carpus.
4	Femur	Horse	There is no third trochanter. Fibula is only a small point projection.
		Ox	Possesses third trochanter. Fibula extends 2/3 the length of tibia.

2. Physical methods

i) General appearance of meat: color, consistency, odour.

S.No	Meat	General appearance of meat		
		Color	Consistency	Odour
1	Chevon	Light red	Very firm	Goaty
2	Mutton	Light dark red	Firm and dense	Ammoniacal
3	Buffalo	Dark red	Firm	-
4	Beef	Red	Fairly firm	-
5	Bullock	Light to dark red	Firm	-
6	Pork	Light red	Very soft	Urine like
7	Veal	Pale to white	Firm	-
8	Horse	Dark red	Soft	-
9	Dog	Dark red	-	-
10	Poultry	White	Firm	-
11	Camel	Red	Fairly firm	-

ii) General characteristics of body fat: color, consistency, quality etc.

S. No.	Fat	General appearance of body fat		
		Colour	Consistency	Quality
1	Chevon	Pure white	-	Practically no intra muscular fat
2	Mutton	White	Hard and firm	Abundant intra muscular fat
3	Buffalo	Pure white	-	-
4	Beef	Yellowish white	Firm	Intra muscular fat
5	Bullock	White to yellow	Firm to lose	-
6	Pork	White	Soft and greasy	Subcutaneous fat deposition intra muscular also
7	Veal	White	Firm	No intra muscular fat
8	Horse fat	Yellow	Soft and greasy	No intra muscular fat
9	Dog fat	White	-	Slight intra muscular fat
10	Poultry fat	Yellow	Loose	Mostly subcutaneous
11	Camel fat	-	-	-

3. Chemical methods

Fat percentage: muscular fat content varies according to the species- mutton13.3%, pork 4.4%, chevon 3.6%, beef 2.6%, carabeef 0.9%.

Myoglobin content: horse flesh contains maximum myoglobin content (0.71%), much higher than the muscle of other animals.

Glycogen content: horse flesh is richer in glycogen as compared to food animals.

Chemistry of fat

S.No.	Characteristics	Species	Value
1	Refractive index of fat	Horse	53.5
		Ox	Less than 40
		Pig	Less than 50
2	Iodine number of fat	Horse	70-85
		Lard	50-70
		Ox	35-46
		Sheep	35-46
3	Carotene content in fat	Buffalo (white)	Absent
		Cow (cream to yellow)	Present
4	Fatty acid analysis of fat (linoleic acid)	Horse	1-2
		Other animal	Less than 0.1

4. Electrophoretic methods

- This method is based on separation of protein by using electrophoresis. The individual extract of protein form bands based on its molecular weight or isoelectric pH.
- Electrophoretic methods have been found to achieve the separation of proteins by their differential migration through a supporting medium under the influence of an electric field.

i) Polyacrylamide disc electrophoresis

- Mitochondrial preparation of goat, sheep, cattle and buffalo meat has been used for particular species of fresh meat which are identified according to the band pattern.

ii) Polyacrylamide-gel-electrophoresis (PAGE)

- After electrophoresis and staining, band pattern is observed for identification.
- It is applicable to meat cooked at less than 80 ^{0}C for 10 mins.

iii) SDS-Page

- Here, proteins run according to their molecular weights.
- The resultant bands can be observed for species specificity.
- Highly useful for cooked meat and meat products.

iv) Iso-electric focusing (IEF)

- It is mainly based on the migration of proteins in a pH gradient.
- The process stops when the surface charges become neutral, at isoelectric point.
- The subsequent fixing makes the protein precipitated and fixed at the same point as bands.
- It is a suitable method for identification of animal species even after cooking at 100 °C.
- Not suitable for frozen meat and closely related meat species.

5. Serological methods

A reaction between soluble antigen and its corresponding specific antibody yields a precipitate. These techniques are simple and can be performed anywhere with little efforts.

i) Precipitation test

- It is also known as ring precipitation test (RPT) in which antigen and antibodies reacts to make a ring.
- If precipitation line forms then it indicates positive test.
- It gives false positive test in closely related species due to cross reactivity.
- In this ring is difficult to observe and difficult in a short period of time.

ii) Double immune-diffusion (DID) test

- This test is extensively used for detection of meat species.
- It is performed in well, punched on agarose gel.
- Buffalo anti-cattle serum and rabbit anti-cattle serum found to be most suitable.
- It is easy and cheap test for identifying raw or heated meat at 80°C.
- It can detect adulteration up to 5%.
- It is time consuming and ineffective for thoroughly cooked meat.

iii) Complement fixation test (CFT)

- Also known agar gel precipitation test (AGID).
- Principle is same as precipitation test but a compliment is used to reproduce the results for longer duration.
- Guinea pig serum as complement and sheep RBCs and rabbit serum used as indicator
- This test can be used both qualitative and quantitative test.
- Adulteration up to 5% and meat cooked at 80°C for less than 10 min can be detected.

iv) Counter immune-electrophoresis (CIE)

- CIE is an immune-diffusion test in which electric voltage is used for acceleration of protein movement.
- In this technique alkaline gel is used which causes electro-osmosis.
- Homologous antibodies and proteins move towards each other and forms a precipitation band.
- It is rapid and more sensitive, can detect one part of species in 300 part of meat;

v) Enzyme-linked immunosorbant assay (ELISA)

- ELISA is an important qualitative immunological tool, not monitored by precipitation.

- Here, antigen-antibody reaction occurs in a monomolecular layer immobilized on an inert surface.
- It is monitored by means of an enzyme chemically bonded to one of the immuno-reagents.
- This is a rapid test and the results are obtained in 2-3 hours.
- The test is very sensitive and can detect even 2% adulteration.

6. Molecular biology methods

DNA based molecular techniques

- Analysis of DNA rather than protein is more useful for species identification due to its stability at high temperature.
- The mitochondrial DNA is more conserved in different species of animals.
- Cytochrome b gene is most commonly targeted for meat identification.
- Mitochondrial 12s rRNA gene with higher precision.

i) Polymerase chain reaction (PCR)

- PCR is a rapid method, we can obtain copies of specific piece of DNA sequence in vitro and it has high specificity and sensitivity.
- PCR amplifies a target DNA sequence, capable of detecting even a single copy from a single cell sample.
- It is a qualitative test for meat species specification.
- Closely related meat species, male and female raw meat can be identified.

ii) Random amplified polymorphic DNA fingerprinting (RAPD)

- Modified PCR- DNA fingerprints are generated in very short time, visualized on gel electrophoresis.
- Prior knowledge of DNA sequence not required but known standard has to run each time.
- DNA extracted from sample amplified with specific primers.
- DNA fragments are visualized by UV trans-illumination.

iii) Species –specific PCR

- In this technique species-specific DNA can be detected in both raw and processed meat samples by targeted amplification of rRNA genes (12, 16, 18 S),
- Actin-multigene, myofibrillar components, cytochrome -b gene.
- Old samples even more than 100 million years can also be identified.

iv) Multiplex PCR

- In this technique many targets are simultaneously amplified which helps in detection of many species in a short period of time.
- Organ meat can also be detected like mixing of duck liver in goose liver.
- Common forward and species –specific reverse primers to nuclear repeated target (5S rDNA gene) is used.

v) PCR– restricted fragment length polymorphism (PCR-RFLP)

Modified PCR: target gene is amplified and resultant PCR product is digested with specific restriction endonuclease enzyme to get a restriction pattern or fingerprints.

- Suitable for identification of even degraded DNA
- First step is extraction of DNA polymerase and specific primers.
- Suitable for very low amount of meat (1mg).
- Faster and more sensitive than DNA hybridization.
- Identification of male and females by using PCR and genomic DNA from meat.
- Not hundred per cent accurate due to some intra-species variability (sheep, turkey and chicken meat).

vi) Forensic informative nucleotide sequencing (FINS)

- Conserved region of gene specific to a species is amplified
- PCR product is cloned, sequenced and analysed.

- 12S rRNA gene sequence analysed for differentiation of beef, buff, mutton and chevon.

vii) Real time PCR

- In this method PCR products are monitored and detected during amplification in the same reaction vessel with the help of fluorescent compounds.
- The technique identifies the product during its amplification.
- In this technique quantification of the meat species may be possible.

❑❑❑

14

Organic and Genetically Modified Meat

What is an Organic Farming

An organic farming is a holistic production management system which promotes agro-ecosystem, health, including biodiversity, biological cycles, and, soil biological activity. It emphasizes to use farm inputs and using cultural, biological, mechanical methods (CAC).

Why should we go for organics

- Makes food taste great
- Free from additives
- Eliminate health risk
- Protect water quality
- Protect future generation's health
- Preserving our livestock
- Preserve topsoil
- Preserve biodiversity

What is an organic meat

- Raising of animal the organic way of handling, the meat so produced is organic.
- Organic meat means that are produced, harvested, preserved and processed as per organic standards.

Raising livestock the organic way

- Provision of conditions to suit health and natural behavior with access to the outdoors, fresh air, water, sunshine, grass and pasture.

- Feeding only organic feed – the dam of animal to be organically raised in last trimester of gestation.
- No offals of any kind in meat, strict vegetarian diet, no plastic pellets as feed, no antibiotics, hormone, urea or manure in feed.
- Animal houses to accord comfort and opportunity to exercise.
- Facilities for onsite inspection.

Indian standards for organic meat production

- For organic meat production animals must be born and raised on an organic farm.
- When organic livestock not available, certification authority may allow to by conventional animals according to following age limits.
  - Two day old chicken for meat production.
  - Piglets up to six weeks after weaning.
  - Calves up to 4 weeks and have been fed mainly a milk diet.
  - Breeding stock may be brought from conventional farms but maximum replacement will be 10 percent.

Breeds and breeding

- Breeds should be chosen which are adapted to local conditions.
- Reproduction techniques should be natural.
- Embryo transfer technologies are not allowed.
- Hormonal treatments are not allowed.
- Use of GMO (genetically modified organisms) not allowed.

Housing

- Animals are not cased, tethered or confined in building without adequate natural ventilation and light.
- Enough space for free movement and kept in appropriate herd size.

Feeding

- Livestock should be fed 100% organically grown feed.
- In some cases 15-20% of total feed could be obtained from conventional farm.
- More than 50% of total feed shall come from the farm itself or produced within region.
- Animals have access to pasture and fresh water.
- Use of synthetic growth promoter, appetizers, preservatives, artificial colouring agents, urea, animal by products to ruminants, solvent extracted oil cakes, pure amino acids, genetically engineered organisms are not allowed.

Animal health

- Natural medicines and methods including homeopathy, ayurvedic medicine and acupuncture shall be emphasized.
- Use of conventional veterinary medicines is allowed when no other alternative is available. If used, the withholding period shall be twice the legally required period.
- Vaccines can be used where the disease is not controlled by management techniques.
- Genetically engineered vaccine are prohibited.

Processed products

- Restriction on use of not more than 55 non organic agricultural products.
- Chemicals like sodium, potassium, calcium citrate, lactic acid are only permitted.
- Nitrite (which prevents the development of botulism) has not been permitted.

Positive effect of organic production in society

- Improve drinking water quality.
- Micro nutrient rich organic foods.
- Achieve rural development generating income and employment.

Negative effect of organic production in society

- Result in decrease in food security in terms of food availability, access, stability.
- Decrease production and increase commodity prices.
- CDC (US) reveals that people eat organic food are prone to attack by new strain of *E. coli* (O157:H7) than rest of population.
- Organic food consumers also face increase risk of illness from toxin produced by fungus.

Positive effect of organic production on meat quality

- Organic meat have better flavour.
- Organic meat give higher guarantee for the absence of chemical residues.
- Better activity of animal reduce abdominal fat and favour muscle development.
- Increase breast percentage in the chicken.
- Organic meat is high in moisture, saturated fatty acid but low in WHC, pH and fat.

Negative Effect of organic production on meat quality

- Lower quality carcass and meat due to low energy supply and growth performance; due to more locomotary activity and uncontrolled environment.
- *Trichnella* and *Salmonella*, etc, are present in organic meat due to lack of prophylactic treatment and outdoor rearing.

Market for organic meat

There is a demand for organic meat and meat products throughout the world. For exporting organic meat and meat products, animals should be grown in their own organic standards.

Distinction between Conventional and Organic Meat

Conventional	Organic
Chemical fertilizers applied for raising fodder	Natural fertilizers applied for raising fodder
Chemical insecticides and pesticides for raising fodder	Biological control for raising fodder
Chemical herbicides to manage weeds.	Crop rotation, weeding by hand
Prophylactic measures to prevent diseases and promotion of growth- Antibiotics, hormones, medications	Prophylactic measures to prevent diseases and promotion of growth-organic feed, access to outdoors, rotational grazing, balanced diet and clean housing

Genetically Modified Meat

Genetically modified animals are raised based on application of molecular biological tools. Biotechnology is the implementation of biological technology to produce or modify products and to manipulate cell genome and functions.

What is transgenic animals

- Transgenic animal refers to an animal in which deliberate modification of the genome is done, which is responsible for inherited characteristics.
- The term transgenic was first used by J.W.Gordon and F.H. Ruddle in 1981.
- Foreign DNA is introduced into the animal, using recombinant DNA technology.
- It must be transmitted through the germ line so that every cell of the animal contains modified genetic material.
- The first successful transgenic animal was mouse followed by rabbits, pigs, sheep, and cattle.

Methods of creation of transgenic animal

1. DNA microinjection

- It is first method that proved to be effective in mammals.

- Process of direct microinjection of chosen gene construct into the pro-nucleus of a fertilized ovum.
- The manipulated fertilized ovum is transferred into oviduct of recipient female.
- The introduced DNA may lead to the under / over expression of certain genes or to the expression of new genes.

Advantages: It is applicable to a wide variety of species.

Disadvantage: The insertion of DNA is a random process. There is a high probability that the introduced gene will not insert itself into a site on the host DNA that will permit its expression.

2. Embryonic stem (ES) cell-mediated gene transfer

- ES cell- mediated gene transfer is the method of choice for gene inactivation, also called **knock-out method.**
- Insertion of the desired DNA sequence into an in-vitro culture of embryonic stem cells.
- These stem cells are then incorporated into an embryo at the blastocyst stage and result is a **chimeric animals**.

3. Retrovirus-mediated gene transfer

- Genetic material is transferred by retrovirus (as a vector) into the cell to increase the probability of expression.
- Transmission of the transgene is possible only if the retrovirus integrates into some of the germ cells.
- Offspring from this methods are chimeric.
- When the transgene has integrated into the germ cells, the so-called germline chimers are then inbred for 10 to 20 generations until homozygous transgenic animals are obtained.
- At these stage embryos carrying the transgene can be frozen and stored for subsequent implantatiom.

Achievements of transgenesis

1. To promote growth and improve the meat quality traits of domestic animal.
2. Average daily gain increased with the supplement of the diet with high level protein.
3. Reduction of body fat and increased diameter of muscle fibre.

In some cattle breeds a gene encoding myostatin, a growth factor that normally inhibit the growth of skeletal muscle cells. Myostatin activity can be blocked by use of transgene that lead to the increase of muscles growth and muscles differentiation.

Introduction of growth-promoting genes into farm animals

Promoter	Gene Coding for	Effect of Trans-genesis
	PIG	
Mouse MT	Bovine GH	Increased growth
	Human GRF	Increased growth
	Human GH	Expression
	Human IGF-I	Expression
Bovine prolactin	Bovine GH	Expression
PEPC	Bovine GH	Increased growth
Mouse albumin	Human GRF	Expression
Human MT	Porcine GH	Increased growth
MSV	Chicken Oncogene C-Ski	Muscle overgrowth or atrophy
	SHEEP	
Mouse MT	Human GH	Integration; expression
	Bovine GH	Integration; expression
	Human GRF	Integration; expression
Ovine MT	Ovine GH	Expression

Purpose	Animal Model	Transgenic Source
Faster growth or leaner meat	Cattle, Swine, Rabbits, Sheep	Growth hormones/factors; Humans, bovine, porcine, rat, Chicken
Altered milk composition (higher protein)	Cattle	Extra coples of casein genes, disruption of lactoglobulin gene
Anti-clotting drug production in milk	Goat	Human antithrombin gene
Faster growth	Atlantic salmon	Growth hormone regulating gene from pacific Chinook salmon and a promoter from ocean pout

□□□

15

National and International Laws for Meat Trade

Meat being a highly perishable commodity requires strict quality control right from slaughter operations till ultimate consumption. The basic objectives of quality control are:

i) Safe guard public health

ii) Monitor product shelf life

iii) Consumer satisfaction

iv) Compliance of regulations

The principles of quality control for meat foods

i) Raw material control

ii) Control of processing operations

iii) Finished product inspection and control

It is very difficult to examine meat and meat products for every pathogenic and spoilage microorganisms. Hence, the following indicator organisms are enumerated to assess their quality:

1. **Total Viable Counts:** These are estimates of mesophiles and psychrophiles and serve as useful indicators of handling history and state of freshness or spoilage of meat. However, if these counts are less, most probable number (MPN) are enumerated.

2. **Coliforms:** These consist of *E. coli* and *Aerobactor aerogenes*. Their presence indicates faecal contamination due to unhygienic handling during or after processing. However, *E. coli* is a better indicator of faecal contamination.

3. **Enterococci:** These are members of faecal streptococci consists of *S. faecalis, S. faecium, S. Bovis, S. Equines*. These organisms

indicate poor hygienic quality of frozen meats and inadequate heat treatment of canned meats.

4. **Other Indicators:** Specific organisms like *Staph. aureus, Salmonella,* Yeast and Mold counts are also important.

Standards in meat Industry

- Regulations are important for quality and pricing.
- A microbial standard is a microbiological criterion that is part of a law, or regulation, mandatory and enforceable by the regulatory agency involved.
- A microbial specification is a microbiological criterion that is applied as a condition of acceptance for a food.
- Quality control departments utilize the reliable methods for establishing the standards.
- A *standard* can be referred as carefully drawn specification with respect to a food product.
- The specifications give comprehensive instructions to ensure process control.
- The compliance of specifications increases the confidence on perishable food items.

Indian laws/regulations

The Indian parliament has recently passed the Food Safety and Standards Act (FSSA) 2006. This act has repealed the following acts/ laws related to meat and meat products.

1. The Prevention of Food Adulteration Act 1954.
2. The Meat Food Products Order 1973.
3. Essential Commodities Act 1955.
4. Consumer Protection Act 1986.
5. Export (Quality Control and Inspection) Act 1963.
6. Foreign Trade Policy for Export of Sheep/Goat/Buffalo.

These acts were to ensure the standards for meat foods and to regulate and monitor the manufacturer, processing, storage, distribution, sale and import to ensure the availability of safe and wholesome food for human consumption. Many of the provisions are adapted in FSSA and some are being revised by Food Safety and Standard Authority of India (FSSAI).

Meat Food Products Order (MFPO)

In 1973, Government of India promulgated an Order to enforce strict quality control on the production and processing of meat food products under Essential Commodities Act 1955

Categories: MFPO, 1973 initially categorises the meat food manufacturers into the following three broad heads on the basis of source of raw meat:

- **Category A**: Includes those manufacturers or licences of meat food products who possess their own slaughterhouse.
- **Category B:** Includes those manufacturers of meat food products who purchase meat from approved slaughterhouse.
- **Category C:** Includes those manufacturers of meat food products, who purchase raw meat from any other source.
- The licence fee for each category differs and is collected every year at the time of renewal of licence.

Bureau of Indian Standards (BIS)

- Established in 1947 as Indian Standard Institution (ISI) as a joint venture of Government of India and Industry took up the responsibility of preparing and promoting the general adoption of standards in the country.
- The erstwhile ISI constituted the Meat and Meat products Sectional Committee, AFDC 18 under the Agricultural and Food Products Division Council in 1958 to prepare Indian Standards for meat industry.
- This committee represents the scientists, technologists, manufacturers, government agencies and consumers.
- The standards are prepared keeping in mind the needs of industry protecting the interests of both producers and consumers and are reviewed periodically.

Food safety and standards Act, 2006

- For implementation/ enforcement, the Food Safety & Standards Authority of India (FSSAI) was constituted on 5.09.2008.

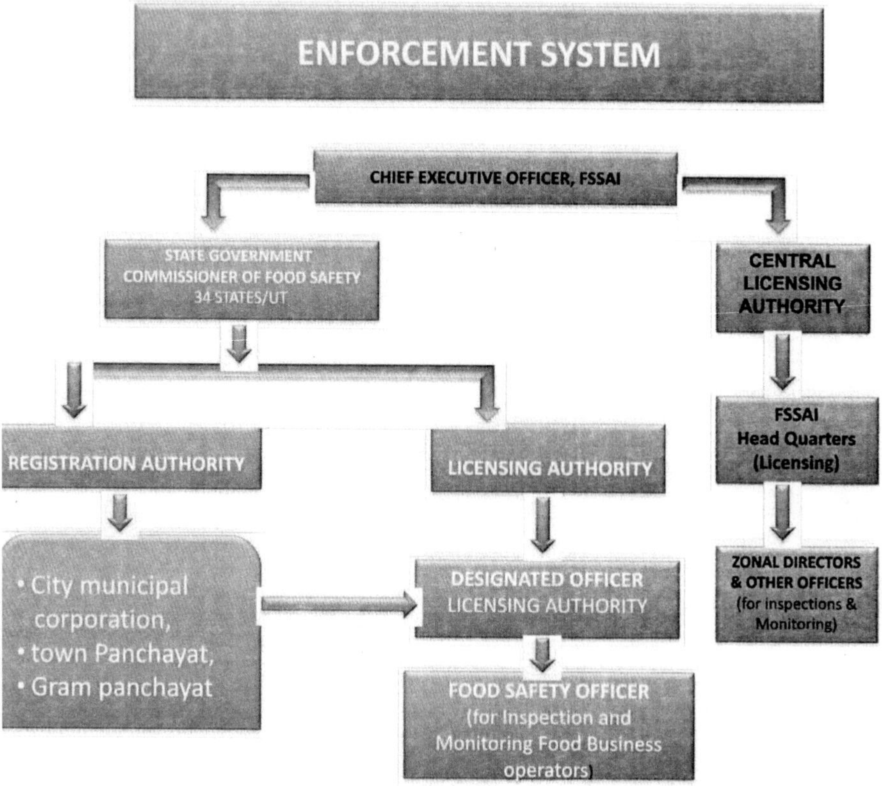

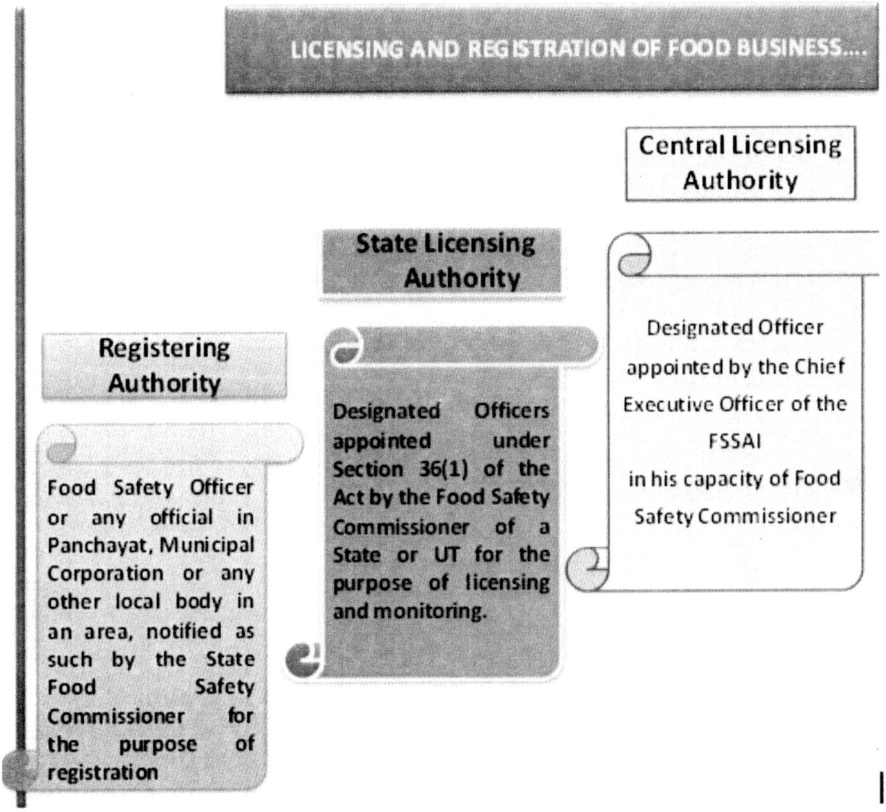

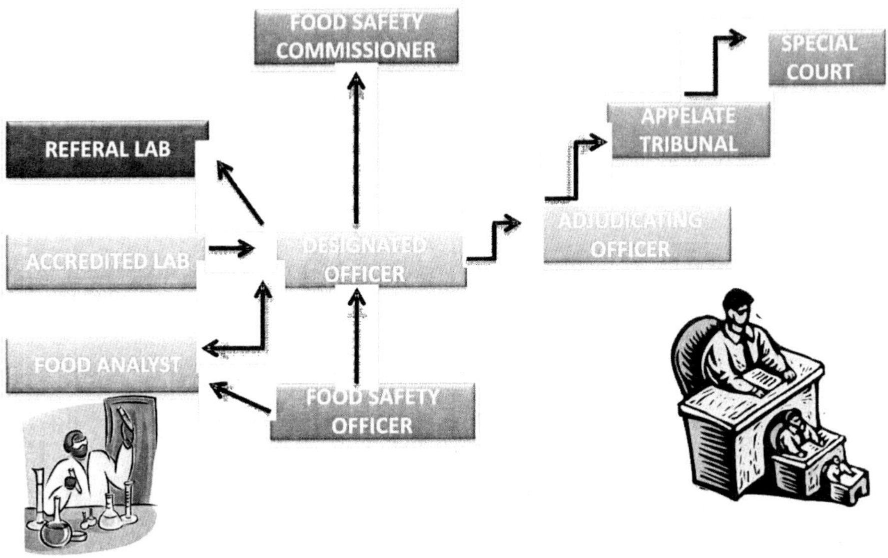

Regulatory Enforcement at State

International laws/regulations/standards

- To meet a country's sanitary and phtyo-sanitary requirements, food must comply with the local laws and regulations to gain market access.
- These laws ensure the safety and suitability of food for consumers in a country.
- The requirements based on adoption of international norms by the Codex Alimentarius Commission (CAC), Good Hygienic Practices (GHP), Good Manufacturing Practices (GMP).
- The major standards governing international food trade is, ISO 9000, now ISO 22000 standard.
- Microbial standards are set by International Committee on Microbial Specification on Foods (ICMSF), and European Economic Community.

ISO 9000 quality management system

The ISO 9000 quality management system was designed to meet the needs of customers and other stakeholders along with statutory and regulatory requirements.

ISO 9000 deals with the fundamentals of quality management systems.

ISO 9001 deals with model for design production installation and servicing.

ISO 9002 deals with model for assurance in production and installation.

ISO 9003 deals with model for quality assurance in final inspection and testing.

ISO 9004 deals with the model for technical administrative and human factor and services.

Benefits of ISO 9000 quality system

- It enables the user to identify and plan task and their method of performance.
- It cuts down the poor quality cost.

- It reduces fire fighting operations and better job satisfaction.
- Marketing advantages , recognition 7 publicity.
- Reduced liability risk.
- Arranging a preliminary audit by an external agency.
- Taking corrective actions on the basis of the external audit team.

ISO 22000 food safety management system

It is a generic food safety management system standard. It defines a set of general food safety requirements that applies to all organization in the food chain.

ISO 22000 can be used by :

- Primary producers (Agriculture aquaculture, horticulture, dairy etc.).
- Food processors and manufacturers.
- Retailers, storage facilities and transporters.
- Hospitality sector- hostels restrooms catering institutes.
- Services providers too food establishments.

Objectives of ISO 22000

- To establish a food safety management system (FSMS).
- To plan and implement a FSMS for your organisation.
- To ensure that product do not cause adverse effect.
- To evaluate your consumers' food safety requirements.
- To export food products and penetrate international markets.
- To demonstrate compliance to all interested parties.

ISO 22000 and HACCP

- Conduct a food safety hazard analysis.
- Identify your critical control points (CCP).
- Establish critical limits for each CCP.

- Develop procedures to monitor CCP.
- To create a food safety record keeping system.
- Validate and verify your system.

National and International standards/specifications on microbiological quality

ICMSF microbial standards for meat

S.No.	Product	Test	n	c	m	M
1.	Carcass meat, before chilling	APC	5	3	10^5	10^6
2.	Carcass meat. chilled	APC	5	3	10^6	10^7
3.	Edible offal, chilled	APC	5	3	10^6	10^7
4.	Carcass meat, frozen	APC	5	3	5×10^5	10^7
5.	Boneless meat, frozen (beef, pork, mutton)	APC	5	3	$5x10^5$	10^7
6.	Comminuted meat, frozen	APC	5	3	10^6	10^7
7.	Edible offal, frozen	APC	5	3	$5x10^5$	10^7
8.	Raw chicken, fresh or frozen	APC	5	3	$5x10^7$	10^7

Where,

- **n** = number of samples to be taken from the lot.
- **c** = number of samples permitted to fail.
- **m** = microbial count below which the sample is considered to be satisfactory.
- **M** = microbial count above which the sample is considered unsatisfactory.

EEC microbial standards for meat

S.No.	Organism	n	c	m	M
1.	Aerobic mesophile (total viable count) bacteria	5	2	$5x10^5$	$5x10^6$
2.	*E.coli*	5	2	$5x10^2$	$5x10^3$
3.	*Cl. perfringens* (sulphite-reducing anaerobes)	5	1	10^2	10^4
4.	Staphylococci	5	1	$5x10^2$	$5x10^3$
5.	Salmonella	5	0	Absence in 25g	

BIS standard for meat and meat products

Food	TPC	*E. coli*	*Salmonella*	*S. aureus*	*Cl. Perfringens*	*Listeria spp*
1	$<10^{3}$/g	Nil /25g	Nil/25g	Nil/25g	Nil/25g	Nil/25g
2	$<10^{5}$	$<10^{2}$	Nil/25g	$<10^{2}$	<30/g	Nil/25g

*Yeast & mould 100/g,

1= Corned beef, Luncheon meat, cooked ham, chopped meat, canned chicken, canned mutton & goat meat

2=Frozen mutton, Goat, Beef & Buffalo meat

BIS standard for chicken sausages

Characteristics	Requirement	
	Uncooked	**Cooked**
Aerobic plate count, per g, Max	10^{6}	10^{3}
Faecal Streptococci, per g, Max	1000	100
Coagulase +ve *S. aureus*, per g, Max	100	10
Faecal coliforms, per g, Max	100	10
Salmonella in 25g	Nil	Nil
Yeast & mould	100	Nil

BIS specification for frozen egg liquid

Parameter	Albumen	Yolk	Whole egg
SPC/gm	20-25 thousand	20-25 thousand	20-25 thousand
Yeast &mould/g	10	10	10
Coliform	10	10	10
Salmonella	Nil	Nil	Nil
Impurities	Nil	Nil	Nil
Solids	11-12	43-45	24-25
Protein	10-10.5	13.5-14	12
Fat	0.02-0.03	27-28	11-11.5
Ash	0.6-0.7	1.5-1.6	0.5-1.0

16

Composition, Quality and Packaging of Egg

Structure of an Egg

1. *Shell:* Outer protective covering- Mainly composed of calcium carbonate. Shell contain numerous minute pores (allows loss of CO_2, moisture and bacterial entry). It contains 3 basic units: (a) Outer cuticle made of keratin, (b) Middle spongy or calcareous layer and (c) Inner mammilary layer.

2. *Shell membrane* - It acts as barrier against bacterial invasion. It has 2 membranes a. Outer and b. Inner thin membrane. Between the 2 layers, air cell is formed at the broad end.

3. *Albumen or White* - 58% of total egg weight, occurs in two layers: (a) Outer thin, (b) Inner thick albumen (c) *Chalazae:* The firm mucin like fibres from thick albumen keeping the yolk in the centre.

4. *Yolk*- 31% of total egg weight, consists of 4 structures: (a) Vitelline membrane, (b) Concentric rings of light and dark yolk material, (c) Latebra (cone like portion extending to the centre of the yolk) (d) Germinal disc (located in the cone of latebra).

Composition of chicken egg

- A large egg weighs about 58 gm of which 11% shell, 58% white and 31% yolk.
- On the basis of interior content 65% white and 35%yolk.
- On commercial breaking yields are 55.57% white and 43-45% yolk.
- The total solid content of albumen ranges from 11 to 13%.

- Egg shell constitutes 11% of egg weight and contains 94% $CaCO_{3,}$ 1% $MgCO_3$, 1% $CaPO_4$ and 4% organic.
- The pH of freshly laid egg albumen is in the range of 7.6-8.5, but increase during storage up to 9.7.

Chemical composition of egg

	Weight	Water (%)	Protein (%)	Fat (%)	Ash (%)	Sugar (%)
Whole egg	100	65.5	11.8	11.0	11.7	0.80
White	58	88.0	11.0	0.2	0.8	1
Yolk	31	48.0	17.5	32.5	2.0	1
Whole egg liquid	89	73.7	12.9	11.5	1.0	1

Important proteins in albumen

Protein	Percentage	Characteristics
Ovalbumen	54	Phosphoglycoprotein
Conalbumen	13	Chelates Fe, Cu, Zn
Ovomucoid	11	Trypsin inhibitor
Lysozyme	3.5	Lyses cell wall
Ovomucin	1.5	Sialoprotein
Flavoprotein	0.8	Binds riboflavin
Ovoinhibitor	0.1	Inhibits proteases
Avidin	0.05	Binds biotin

Nutritive value of egg

- Eggs contain about 65 per cent water and are rich source of protein that is of high biological value.
- An egg contains 6-7 gm protein, containing all the essential amino acids.
- An egg also contains 5-6 gm fat, readily digestible, contains less than 0.4g CHO, 180 in calories, can be used in low calorie diet.
- Eggs are important source of essential fatty acids oleic, linoleic, linolinic acid.
- Rich in Iron, Phosphorus, trace minerals, the fat-soluble vitamins A, D, E, K and many of the water-soluble B vitamins.

- The egg is potent source of vitamin D but low in calcium and devoid of vitamin C.
- Egg yolk is high in cholesterol 250-270 mg.
- Fat soluble vitamins are more in yolk, however, water soluble are present in both white and yolk.

Quality of egg

Interior and exterior quality of egg along with size and weight is important for quality assessment and grading of egg. Some of these quality aspects which can be easily measured are briefly described.

Exterior quality

1. *Shape and structure:* Shape is measured by shape index. Width and length of egg is measured by slide callipers.

   $$\text{Shape Index} = \frac{\text{Width} \times 100}{\text{Length}}$$

   Chicken eggs have a shape index of 74. Oval shape is considered to be normal, if not oval it is called as unusual shape.

2. *Soundness of Shell:* In a sound egg the shell will be intact and unbroken. Abnormalities can be :

   Checked - there may be slight cracks but not leaking

   Leaking - oozing of internal contents

   Smashed - crashing of an area

3. *Shell cleanliness:* The different categories may be- clean, slightly stained, moderately stained, dirty.

4. Shell thickness: Can be measured with the help of paper thickness micrometer or slide calipers.

5. *Air cell*: The depth of air cell is a rough indication of the age of the egg and there is a relation between this depth and internal quality. Air cell may be :

   a) Large –exceeds 6 mm in depth.

   b) Running –moving between two shell members caused by rough handling.

   c) Ringed –very large, sharply defined with grey or brown edges.

6. *Specific gravity:* Is measured by dipping in solutions of different specific gravities called "brine floatation technique". Brine solutions of 1.062 -1.102 specific gravity is taken with an interval of 0.004.

7. *Shell percent:* weight of shell alone is taken and then its percent is calculated as :

   Weight of shell/weight of egg x 100.

Interior quality of egg

1. *Albumen*: Albumen index is an indicator of the albumen quality with a maximum value of 0.1. In practice the quality of egg white is judged by the degree of movement of the yolk and definition of its outline.

   Albumen index = Height of albumen/Average width of albumen.

   Height of the albumen is measured with the help of tripod micrometer.

2. *Yolk:* The judgement of internal quality is mainly based on the visibility, movement and shape of the yolk. Yolk index is also an indicator of the yolk quality with a maximum value of 0.5.

   Yolk index = Height of yolk/average width of yolk.

Natural defence in egg

1. Membrane layers under the shell.
2. Degree of inherent impermeability of shell.
3. A group of antibiotic substance in albumen.
4. Antibacterial effect due to raised pH of albumen.

Physico-chemical alterations during storage

The rate of physico-chemical changes in the egg depends upon the time and temperature of holding, the relative humidity and the composition of the atmosphere.

1. Drying of surface, keratin shrinks, pores increases- facilitates entry and exit of microbes and gases.

2. Loss of moisture and cooling of egg causes internal shrinkage and increase air cell.
3. Break down of carbonic acid-form carbon dioxide-pH increases, albumen looses firmness.
4. Internal migration of water from albumen to yolk causes flabby yolk, may rupture.
5. Loss of normal firmness of egg white, becomes watery.
6. Outer membrane becomes fragile, more susceptible to microbial growth.

Steps in microbial spoilage

1. Penetration of shell
2. Colonization
3. Overpowering antibacterial factors in albumen.
   - Micro organisms penetrate through shell pores, grow in shell membrane, in the egg white, or in the yolk.
   - More spoilage of egg is due to bacteria than by molds.

Common types of spoilage of egg

Type of Rot / Odour	Changes in Egg	Caused by
Green rot	Albumen becomes green	*Pseudomonas fluorescens*
Black rot	Blackening of yolk with "fecal odour"	*Proteus* sp.
	Green coloured albumen but yolk is black with "cabbage odour"	*Pseudomonas*
Red rot	Albumen stained red throughout yolk surrounded by custard like material	*Serratia* sp.
Fungal rot ("whiskers")	Pink spots on egg contents	*Sporotrichium*
	Black spots on contents	*Cladosporium*
	Yellow or Green spots on contents	*Penicillium*

Packaging of eggs

Eggs are provided with natural package-like shell and shell membrane. However, the egg is an extremely fragile product and even with the best handling, serious losses can result from shell damage.

- Proper packaging of eggs protects them against dirt and reduces damage during storage, transport and distribution.
- The packaging materials must be clean and they should provide maximum cushioning effect.
- Egg should be properly cleaned and graded prior to packaging.
- Eggs of different grades are packaged separately.
- Eggs are kept with broad end up in moulded paper or plastic filler flats.
- In developed countries, packed eggs are transported in the refrigerated van.

Grain by-products

- Packing eggs with rice husks, chopped straw in basket or crate decreases the shell damage.
- This kind of packaging is suitable for short distance transport.

Filler Trays

- Moulded pulp or plastic filler flats are most commonly used for packaging of eggs.
- Fillers can be covered with plastic films for final sale.
- Plastic transparent fillers allow easy counting and inspection of eggs without handling.
- Commonly filler flats consist of 6 rows of five eggs (total 30).
- The flats are stacked in wooden, plastic or cardboard boxes/ cartons in shipping containers.
- Cardboard boxes to contain 360 or 210 eggs in filler flats are used in rail transport.

Retail packages

- Eggs can also be packed for retail sale with 2-12 nos.
- Two rows of 6, two rows of 3 or one row of 6 eggs are the usual retail packs.
- Small cases made of paperboard, wood pulp, or plastic covered with plastic film.
- Polystyrene cases provide cushioning and protection against odours and moisture.
- Small cases are good for retailers to handle and customers to inspect the eggs.

Overwrapping

- Polyethylene, cellophane, or other transparent strong films are used.
- These films should be impervious to gases and moisture.

Labelling

- Contain information about the size, weight and grade description - AA, A or B.
- Labels may indicate the producer, date, how to store and their expiry date.

17

Preservation and Processing of Egg

Preservation of Shell Egg

Egg meant for consumption should have clean and intact shell, good internal quality and desirable taste and flavour. This can be achieved by adopting better methods of assembly, cleaning, grading, preservation, packing, storage, transportation and distribution of eggs.

Proper handling practices for eggs

- Collection 3-4 times /day to avoid dirts and breakage.
- After collection hold at 15°C at 70-80% relative humidity.
- Pack in filler flats broad end up, bulk packing in fibre cartons.
- Rapid movement through marketing to avoid time lapse.

Egg cleaning

- Earlier days dry cleaning with abrasive cloth were practiced.
- Only dirty eggs are subjected to washing.
- Washing in warm water with detergent effective for dirty shells.
- A temperature of 10-15°C is ideal for cleaning.
- Immerse in water not for more than 3-4 min
- After washing eggs should be dried immediately.
- It reduces the bacterial load on the shell surface and improves the appearance.

1. Lime water treatment

- Lime water is prepared by boiling 0.5kg of quick lime in 1 litre of water.

- Next day take supernatant, add 2.5 litres of water and filter through muslin cloth.
- Keep eggs in this solution for 24 hours then dried and stacked in filler flats.
- Eggs can be kept for 2-3 months in good condition at ambient temperature.

2. Water glass method

- A 10% solution of sodium silicate is prepared in hot water and allowed to cool.
- Eggs are immersed completely in the solution and kept in a cool place.
- Eggs are usually punctured before boiling to avoid the breakage and for easy peeling.

3. Coating with oil

- Coating oil form a thin film on the shell, sealing the pores.
- It should be done within 1st few hours, because loss of CO_2 and moisture is more during this period.
- It can be done by dipping the eggs in edible oil, or by spraying the oil.
- The eggs are immersed only for a moment and the excess oil is allowed to drain.
- Oiling is not a substitute for refrigeration and eggs must be held at a low temperature.
- This can safeguard the quality of albumen for 7 days.

4. Thermostabilization

- Immersing shell eggs in hot water at 55°C for 15 minutes and cooled under tap water.
- This treatment tend to coagulate the albumin and block the pores in egg shell
- Treated eggs remain edible for 3 to 4 weeks even during summer months.

5. Cold Storage

- This is the best method for commercial storage.
- For short period of 2 to 3 months, eggs can be stored at 10-12°C at RH 60-70%.
- A temperature of 0°C and RH of 80-85% for storage of eggs for 5-8 months.
- Temperature should be above -2°C to prevent freezing and cracking of shell.
- Similarly, the R.H. of cold store should not exceed 85% to prevent mold growth.
- Oil coating prior to cold storage further enhance the keeping quality.

Liquid egg preservation

It is mandatory to pasteurize egg liquids to destroy all the pathogenic microbes including *Salmonella* spp. and to reduce spoilage organisms as much as possible before dehydration. Pasteurization of egg white is more difficult due to its instability in heat, at high pH.

Pasteurization of egg liquid

1. *Lactic acid with aluminium sulphate-* One ounce (1 oz) of aluminium sulphate mixed in 1lb of 25% lactic acid and added @ of 0.65% in liquid egg. Then egg content is heated at 62°C for 3.5 to 4.0 min. Lactic acid is added to reduce pH to 6.6-7.0, aluminium sulphate to protect conalbumen.
2. *Heat with hydrogen peroxide-* Egg product pH is maintained at normal range and heated to 52-53°C for 1.5 min. A 10% solution of hydrogen peroxide is added into liquid egg at 0.08%. After cooling, catalase is added to neutralize hydrogen peroxide.
3. *Ultra pasteurization.* Heating at 70-72°C for 30 sec followed by aseptic packaging. Shelf-life about one month at 4°C.

Time temperature requirements for pasteurization of different liquid egg products

Egg products	Temperature (°C)	Time (min)
Albumen	57	3.5
Whole eggs (plain)	60	3.5
Salted whole egg (2-10%)	63	3.5
Sugared whole egg (2-12%)	61	3.5
Plain yolk	61	3.5
Sugared yolk (2-10%)	63	3.5

Desugarization

- To prevent Mailard reaction to form brown, off odour compound.
- By removing the glucose in the egg by fermentation using bacteria (*Acrobactor aerogenes*), yeast.
- An enzyme system comprised of glucose oxidase and catalase.

Preparation of egg mélange

- Washing of eggs and breaking them individually in cups by hand or machine.
- Collection of contents as whole liquid, albumen or yolk.
- Homogenization, filtration, desugarization, pasteurization.
- Filtration is done to remove chalazae, vitelline membrane and shell particles, if any.

Freezing of egg liquid

- Whole egg, egg white and yolk are frozen separately depending on the end use.
- Process consists of breaking eggs, homogenization to pasteurization.
- Blast freezing (-30 to -40 °C) in bulk containers and low density polyethylene bags.
- Freezing of egg yolk below -21°C cause gelatinization, can be prevented by adding 0.02-0.03 % pepsin or 0.05 % trypsin.

Egg processing

Reason for egg processing

1. Utilization of surplus eggs.
2. Value addition.
3. Good export value.
4. Easy to handle & transport.
5. Climatic condition.
6. Space saving.
7. Pharmaceutical advantages.

Products of egg processing

Powders from egg white, egg yolk and whole egg.

Other products: lysozyme, avidin, shell membrane, shell powder, lecithin.

Drying

- Dried egg products from albumen, yolk and whole egg depending on their usages.
- If properly dried, they have quality comparable to that of shell eggs.

Advantages of dried egg products

1. Storage cost and space saving.
2. Transportation cost less.
3. Easy to handle.
4. No bacterial growth.
5. Good uniformity
6. Use in new convenience food.

Preparation of whole egg powder

- Methods of egg drying are spray drying, pan drying, belt drying and freeze drying.

- Spray drying is most commonly used for whole egg power, albumen or yolk power.
- Here small droplets of liquid eggs are produced by atomizing and pass through a hot air chamber.
- Because of very rapid evaporation, egg liquid spray is converted into fine powder instantly.

Inspection & cleaning of egg
(detergent wash at 40°C for 3 min)
↓
Breaking and inspection
↓
Homogenization and filtration
↓
Pasteurization at 62.5°C for 3.5 min
(Plate heat exchanger)
↓
Desugarization (Glucose-oxidase or Yeast)
↓
Repasteurization
↓
Spray drying (4-5% moisture, Inlet 160°C & outlet 60°C)
↓
Vacuum drying to reduce moisture to 2 % at 60°C for 2-3 h
↓
Packaging in cans with nitrogen or flexible pouches
↓
Storage
(6 months without N_2 and 12 months with N_2)

Flow diagram for preparation of whole egg powder

Yield of dried egg products

About 4 kg of whole egg liquid, 8 kg of albumen and 2.2 kg of yolk will yield one kg of respective dried egg products.

Albumen flakes

- Dried product prepared from the albumen by pan drying method.
- The edible food grade flake is prepared from fresh, wholesome eggs.

- Albumen must be pasteurized at 54-56°C for 3 min before drying.
- The product is used in the preparation of angel cake, candies, and confectionaries.
- Low grade eggs can be used for non-edible albumen flakes for industrial use.

Preparation of albumen flake

Fresh eggs
↓
Washings (hypochlorite, 40°C, 3 min)
↓
Drying of eggs
↓
Breaking and separation of albumen
↓
Homogenization
↓
Desugaring (0.5% yeast, 12 hrs, 30°C)
↓
Pasteurization (62.5°C, 3-5 min)
↓
pH adjust to 6.6 (by 10% citric acid)
↓
Drying
↓
Packing and storage
(6 months at room temperature)

BIS standard for albumen flake and whole egg powder

Parameter	Albumen flake	Whole egg powder
Moisture (%)	7.1 or 8.0	2
Protein (%)	49.8	45
Fat (%)	0.4	38
*pH	6.93	7.9
Solubility (%)	80-87	85
TPC/g	5.6×10^4	7.5×10^4
Y&M/g	100	50
Coliform/g	100	100

Yolk granules

- The egg yolk is homogenized, filtered to remove vitelline membrane.
- Pasteurized, whipped and sprayed on a perforated belt passing through a heated chamber.
- The dried foam produced is then crushed to desired granulation.
- Used in sponge cake, doughnuts and cookies for its excellent properties.

Packaging of egg products

- All the dried egg products are hygroscopic and sensitive to oxidation.
- The package should protect dehydrated egg products against moisture and O_2 entry.
- Metal cans with N_2 the egg powder has shelf-life up to one year at room temperature.
- Laminated pouches made up of paper/foil/PE flushed with nitrogen.
- Glass containers, if used, should be amber coloured to minimize the oxidation.

❏❏❏